$21·30B5

San...

Studies in Sa...

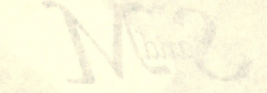

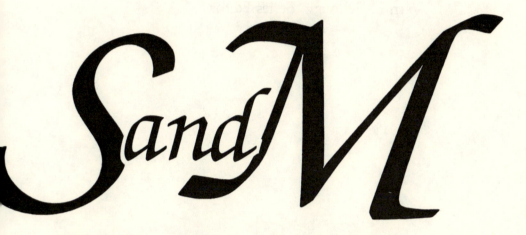

S and M

Studies in Sadomasochism

edited by Thomas Weinberg
and G. W. Levi Kamel

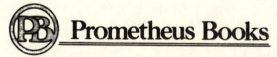

Prometheus Books

700 East Amherst St. Buffalo, New York 14215

New Concepts in Human Sexuality
Vern L. Bullough, Series Editor

Published 1983 by Prometheus Books
700 East Amherst Street, Buffalo, New York 14215

Library of Congress Catalog Number: 83-61030

ISBN: 0-87975-218-1 (Cloth)
0-87975-230-0 (Paper)

Printed in the United States of America

To our mothers,
Rose Lieberberg Weinberg and Mary Louise Hanna Kamel,
with love

Contents

SCENES: S&M INTERACTION

STRUCTURES: THE SOCIAL ORGANIZATION OF S&M

SYNTHESIS: DEVELOPING A SEXOLOGY OF SADOMASOCHISM

Foreword

Sadism and masochism have usually been looked upon by therapists as individual psychopathologies. This perspective gives a distorted view of a widespread phenomenon by ignoring the sociological and cultural factors that encourage and support the existence of sadomasochism. This book will help the therapist, the researcher, and the general reader reach beyond the prevailing narrow and myopic views.

Though history abounds with examples of sadism and masochism, the terms themselves were first coined by the medical forensic specialist Richard von Krafft-Ebing, whose *Psychopathia Sexualis* went through many editions in the last two decades of the nineteenth century. Almost immediately, behavior was defined to fit into the definitions, and what might have been regarded as merely eccentric behavior became a psychopathology. This is best evidenced by the source of Krafft-Ebing's definitions.

Sadism, for example, received its name from the novels and personal life of the Marquis de Sade (1740–1814). Krafft-Ebing defined it as the creation of sexual pleasures in one's self through acts of cruelty or bodily punishments that were inflicted upon others, observed being inflicted upon others, or even at times inflicted on oneself. This last part impinged upon the definition of masochism, a term he coined from the novels and lifestyle of the historian Leopold von Sacher-Masoch (1836–1895). Krafft-Ebing described it as the sexual feeling resulting from being controlled or dominated by the will of a person, or being treated by this person as by a master, of being humiliated and abused. Sacher-Masoch was not defined as ill in his lifetime, and though de Sade was accused of excessive debauchery and fined, his later confinement was for political reasons rather than for any overt sexual activity.

Though sadism and masochism became psychopathologies through the efforts of Krafft-Ebing, they are also forms of social behavior, since they

9

involve relations between or among individuals. Thus, the relationships among these individuals, and the social meanings underlying such things as dominance and submission, aggression and passivity, masculinity and femininity, must also be investigated. In addition, we need to explore how such patterns emerge in the first place and what elements in our society encourage or discourage sadomasochism. Paul Gebhard has argued that sadomasochism "is embedded in our culture since our culture operates on the basis of dominance-submission relationships, and aggression is socially valued" (Gebhard, 1969: 77). That is a strong statement backed up by some of the findings in the early Kinsey studies. Kinsey, for example, found that one in eight females and one in five males were aroused by sadomasochistic stories (Gebhard, 1969: 79).

In the face of the realities of human life, each of us has known an almost infantile helplessness. One way of coping is to trust in a God who in the Christian tradition has often been portrayed as both wanting and desiring the humiliation and/or suffering of his people. Sometimes this tradition almost approaches masochism as, for example, when Pope John Paul began to recover from an attempted assassination, he reported that he had regarded his own sufferings as an offering to his Church and to the world. In this respect he was observing a long tradition dating at least from the Old Testament sufferings of Job and carrying through to the New Testament sufferings of Jesus. This ideology became incorporated into Christianity through the Christian ascetics of the fourth and fifth centuries.

Inevitably, it has long been permissible in our culture to achieve pleasure, even to the point of orgasm, either through giving or receiving punishment. In fact, it has not only been permitted, it has become part of a revered tradition. Therapists or counselors who ignore this long tradition cannot really help their clients. To look upon sadomasochism as a deviance or psychopathology is not enough; we must also take into account the fact that it reflects a deep-seated ambivalence about sexuality in our own society.

Once we come to terms with the widespread tradition of sadomasochism, we see it everywhere: in the gothic novels that so many women seem to love to read; in the Mickey Spillane mysteries that appeal to the macho male, even in the John Wayne movies. Here is the importance of the essays collected by Weinberg and Kamel. They help to break sadomasochism from the narrow confines in which both scholarly study and general public attitudes have placed it. It is widespread; it has a long history in our society. For a time in this country we tried to ban the writings of the Marquis de Sade and Leopold von Sacher-Masoch. One of the consequences of refusing to recognize such phenomena was the shock and surprise with which many of us received the news of the holocaust, or the denials we made about the existence of prison brutality, or the calloused and indifferent treatment we extended to minorities in our own country. Only by coming to terms with the existence of sadomasochism in its many forms can we begin to understand.

Then, if we as a society feel that this is the kind of behavior we do not want to encourage, we might think about some of the causal factors, if such can be identified. To ignore sadomasochism, however, is to ignore life itself; to understand the way society operates we really have to understand human behavior in all its forms. I commend the following studies to you for this reason. The collection is long overdue.

Vern L. Bullough

REFERENCE

Gebhard, Paul H., "Fetishism and Sadomasochism," pp. 71–80 in Jules H. Masserman, ed., *Dynamics of Deviant Sexuality*. New York: Grune & Stratton, 1969.

Preface

The idea for a book on the social aspects of sexual sadomasochism grew out of a series of discussions between the editors that began several years ago when we first met at the University of California, San Diego. Both of us had published papers on this subject independently; we knew of each other, but only by reputation. Our discovery that we were to be office mates was the happy and fortuitous circumstance that led to this collaboration. We found our perspectives on S&M to be quite similar: while not totally eschewing psychoanalytic notions, our emphasis was nevertheless on sadomasochism as *social behavior*. We recognized a real need to develop sociological points of view that would help to fill a large void in the literature on sadomasochism.

The selections in this volume have been chosen to emphasize a viewpoint that only recently has been represented in the professional literature, and even then it has been given sparce attention. In fact, in developing this anthology we have felt the need to include previously unpublished material. We made a very careful and considered decision not to reproduce the standard psychoanalytic essays, since they form the bulk of the writing on sadomasochism and are freely accessible. However, we have been careful to acknowledge their importance in building a theory of sadomasochism. To that end, the classic perspectives of Richard von Krafft-Ebing, Sigmund Freud, and Havelock Ellis are outlined in the first section, entitled "Statements: Classic Perspectives on Sadomasochism." Their importance is further documented in our own essay, "S&M: An Introduction to the Study of Sadomasochism." It is interesting to note that even in the works of these authors, the origins of sadomasochism are attributed to cultural expectations of masculine and feminine behavior.

We would like to acknowledge here the interest and encouragement of several colleagues in this project. Vern L. Bullough has been especially

13

supportive of the book. He contributed much more than just the Foreword; he was also instrumental in helping us place it with a publisher. Jack D. Douglas, Gerhard Falk, John Johnson, and Martha S. Magill were generous with their time and suggestions. We are also indebted to Steven L. Mitchell, our editor at Prometheus Books, for his insights and support in the production of this volume.

Thomas S. Weinberg   G. W. Levi Kamel
Buffalo, NY   La Jolla, CA

STATEMENTS
CLASSIC PERSPECTIVES
ON
SADOMASOCHISM

Thomas S. Weinberg and G. W. Levi Kamel

S&M: An Introduction to the Study of Sadomasochism

WHAT IS SADOMASOCHISM?

"Sadomasochism" (S&M) is a combined term that has traditionally been used for the giving and receiving of pain for erotic gratification. As we shall see, however, such a simple definition is inadequate for describing what is really a very complex type of behavior. "Sadism" and "masochism" were first used in some consistent scientific way by the psychoanalyst Richard von Krafft-Ebing. In *Psychopathia Sexualis,* which first appeared in 1885, Krafft-Ebing defined sadism as "the experience of sexual [*sic*] pleasurable sensations (including orgasm) produced by acts of cruelty, bodily punishment afflicted on one's own person or when witnessed by others, be they animals or human beings." He went on to say that "it may also consist of an innate desire to humiliate, hurt, wound or even destroy others in order thereby to create sexual pleasure in one's self" (Krafft-Ebing, 1965: 53). Krafft-Ebing pointed out that sadism occurred frequently among the "sexual perversions" but he further noted that lovers and young married couples often engaged in some sort of "horseplay," teasing, biting, pinching, and, wrestling "just for fun." Thus, even the roots of extreme displays of sadism were to be found in normal sexual activity. "The transition from these atavistic manifestations, which no doubt belong to the sphere of physiological sexuality, to the most monstrous acts of destructions of the consort's life can be readily traced," he maintained (p. 53). The term *sadism* itself is derived from the Marquis de Sade, a French nobleman and writer who lived during the eighteenth and early nineteenth centuries. Many of de Sade's novels and stories, including *Justine* and *Juliette,* equate cruelty, pain, and humiliation with sexual pleasure.

Krafft-Ebing derived the term *masochism* from the name of Leopold von Sacher-Masoch, whose novels, such as *Venus in Furs,* reflected his personal erotic preoccupation with pain, humiliation, and submission. By "masochism," Krafft-Ebing meant,

> a peculiar perversion of the psychical sexual life in which the individual affected, in sexual feeling and thought, is controlled by the idea of being completely and unconditionally subject to the will of a person of the opposite sex; of being treated by this person as by a master, humiliated and abused. This idea is colored by lustful feeling; the masochist lives in fantasies, in which he creates situations of this kind and often attempts to realize them (p. 86).

Krafft-Ebing's description of masochism is much more detailed and broader than his definition of sadism. He defines masochism not only in terms of the receiving of pain; but also, and most importantly, he recognizes the centrality of fantasy and the nonphysical aspects of dominance and submission to sadomasochistic relationships.

Sigmund Freud, Krafft-Ebing's contemporary, also wrote extensively on sadism and masochism. Like Krafft-Ebing, Freud recognized the existence of sadism in "the normal individual." "The sexuality of most men," he wrote,

> shows an admixture of aggression, of a desire to subdue, the biological significance of which lies in the necessity for overcoming the resistance of the sexual object by actions other than *mere* courting. Sadism would then correspond to an aggressive component of the sexual instinct which has become independent and exaggerated and has been brought to the foreground by displacement (Freud, 1938: 569).

Although Freud and Krafft-Ebing felt that sadism, in its less extreme forms, was understandable in terms of normal male sexuality, they had a much more difficult time in accepting the possible normalcy of masochism, at least among men. Freud considered masochism to be "further removed from the normal sexual goal than its opposite. It may even be doubted whether it ever is primary and whether it does not more often originate through transformation from sadism" (1938: 569). Krafft-Ebing was less explicit than Freud, but a careful reading of *Psychopathia Sexualis* leaves the reader with little doubt that he considered passivity to be less natural for men (but perhaps not for women) than sexual aggression. He writes, "by this perversion his [the male's] sexual instinct is often made more or less insensible to the normal charms of the opposite sex—incapable of a normal sexual life—psychically impotent" (Krafft-Ebing, 1965: 86).

Unlike Krafft-Ebing, Freud saw sadism and masochism as being two forms of the same entity, and he noted that they were often found in the same person:

He who experiences pleasure by causing pain to others in sexual relations is also capable of experiencing pain in sexual relations as pleasure. A sadist is simultaneously a masochist, though either the active or the passive side of the perversion may be more strongly developed in him and thus, represent his preponderant sexual activity (Freud, 1938: 570).

Freud's observation is verified by a number of writers whose articles appear in the present collection. Andreas Spengler finds that a majority of the male sadomasochists he studied defined themselves as "versatile," a definition that made it easier for them to adapt to a variety of partners. Pat Califia, an avowed "sadist," nevertheless reports that she occasionally enjoys taking the masochistic role; and G. W. Levi Kamel points out in his article on gay "leathersex" that "the most exciting S has also served as an M, and the best M is capable of the S role. It is common for an S to have once been an M almost exclusively, and most leathermen begin their sexual lives as slaves" (Kamel, 1980: 183).

Havelock Ellis claimed in *Studies in the Psychology of Sex* that the distinction made between sadism and masochism is artificial. He argued that this division does not correspond with reality and that "sadism and masochism may be regarded as complementary emotional states; they can not be regarded as opposed states" (Ellis, 1942, Vol. 1, Part 2: 159).

Ellis narrowed the definition of sadomasochism used by Krafft-Ebing and Freud; he made reference to "pain" rather than "cruelty." Erotically-motivated pain was, for Ellis, the essence of sadomasochism. He preferred the term "algolagnia," which refers specifically to the connection between sexual excitement and pain, to "sadism" and "masochism." In an important modification of Freud and Kraft-Ebing, Ellis not only rejected the idea that sadomasochism was based upon cruelty, but, most importantly, he also believed that *much of this behavior was actually motivated by love*:

When we understand that it is pain only, and not cruelty, that is the essential in this group of manifestations we begin to come nearer to their explanation. The masochist desires to experience pain, but he generally desires that it should be inflicted in love; the sadist desires to inflict pain, but in some cases, if not in most, he desires that it should be felt as love (Ellis, 1942, Vol. 1, Part 2: 160).

Ellis also noted that "sadists" limit their "love of pain" to sexual situations—an important point that is taken up by some of the writers in the present book—and that the sadist is concerned with the sexual pleasure of the "victim." In fact, he wrote, "the sadist by no means wishes to exclude the victim's pleasure, and may even regard that pleasure as essential to his own satisfaction" (1942, Vol. 1, Part 2; 166). In this work, Ellis foreshadowed

later writers who viewed sadomasochistic situations in terms of social interaction; he noted that sadists do take into account the responses of their
masochists. Yet, in a number of important respects, Ellis failed to understand the essence of S&M as a *social behavior*. First of all, he saw the masochist as essentially a passive participant in the situation. He even referred to
the masochist as a "victim." Actually, however, S&M scenarios are *willingly
and cooperatively* produced; more often than not it is the *masochist's* fantasies that are acted out. Many S&Mers claim, therefore, that the masochist, rather than the sadist, is really in control during a sadomasochistic
episode. The partners jointly limit their mutual activities and these restric-
tions are rarely exceeded. Sadists who are known to disregard previously
agreed upon limits are avoided and quickly find themselves without partners.

Ellis missed the essence of S&M in another way. Although the concept
of cruelty was correctly eliminated from his definition, Ellis's concomitant
limitation of sadomasochism to pain indicates that he knew very little about
what actually happens during S&M scenes. Much S&M involves very little
pain. Rather, many sadomasochists prefer acts such as verbal humiliation
or abuse, cross-dressing, being tied up (bondage), mild spankings where no
severe discomfort is involved, and the like. Often, it is the notion of being
helpless and subject to the will of another that is sexually titillating. It is the
illusion of violence, rather than violence itself, that is frequently arousing to
both sadists and masochists. At the very core of sadomasochism is not pain
but the idea of control—dominance and submission. Krafft-Ebing, of
course, knew this. Nevertheless, both he and Freud still considered sadomasochism to be a "perversion." One of the important contributions Ellis
made was to avoid using that term when writing about S&M. In this regard,
he seems more objective than a number of other psychoanalytically-oriented
writers. Both Frank Caprio (1955) and Wilhelm Stekel (1965), for example,
viewed sadomasochism solely as an individual psychopathology. Their
work was confined to the presentation and psychiatric analysis of case
histories.

In 1969, anthropologist Paul Gebhard published what was to become a
classic article on "Fetishism and Sadomasochism," which represented a real
advance in the study of S&M. Gebhard emphasized that this behavior
occurs within a cultural context:

> Sadomasochism is embedded in our culture since our culture operates
> on the basis of dominance-submission relationships, and aggression is
> socially valued. Even our gender relationships have been formulated in
> a framework conducive to sadomasochism: the male is supposed to be
> dominant and aggressive sexually and the female reluctant or sub-
> missive (p. 77).

Gebhard's belief that sexual aggressiveness and passivity were a product of culture rather than biology represented a significant break from the physiologically-motivated theories of Krafft-Ebing and Freud. Having rooted sadomasochism firmly in culture, Gebhard went on to discuss it as a social behavior. He noted at least four features of this behavior that are directly relevant to understanding S&M as a social phenomenon. First, he discussed the prevalence of S&M in literate societies. Second, he noted the symbolic nature of S&M. Third, he implicitly couched sadomasochism in terms associated with interaction (i.e., interaction between sadist and masochist) and context (emphasizing the importance of social milieu). Finally, and perhaps most insightfully, Gebhard conceptualized S&M activity as scripted behavior.

Gebhard's work illustrates the complexity of sadomasochism. It is not merely a manifestation of individual mental illness, nor is it definable in a single sentence. S&M is, most of all, subcultural social behavior. The variations and "richness" of this subculture, with its own special set of norms and values, language, justifications, even publications and formally structured organizations, are amply described in many of the selections in this volume. Sadomasochism is a sexual lifestyle, one to which notions of dominance and submission are central. It is characterized by socially produced and shared fantasies. For many devotees, sadomasochism is play; it is recreational.

WHY SHOULD WE STUDY SADOMASOCHISM?: S&M AS SOCIAL BEHAVIOR

The importance of devoting serious study to sadomasochism lies in the social nature of this behavior. If, as Paul Gebhard suggested, S&M has its basis in the culture of the larger society, then an examination of this behavior should help us to better understand certain selected aspects of that culture. In a subculture involving S&M, where behavior often takes "extreme" forms, the cultural assumptions underlying human action should be more visible and explicit than is the case in the larger society. In the sadomasochistic world many of the conventional niceties, which normally obscure motives and interests, are stripped away. Hence, the microcosm of interrelationships and social meanings surrounding, for example, dominance and submission, aggression and passivity, and masculinity and femininity should be more amenable to study than they usually are within the larger culture. It is probably not inaccurate to say that what we assume to be "normal" configurations of these qualities are neither normal, inevitable, nor immutable. We find, for example, that in the world of the sadomasochist, there is nothing "abnormal" about a male being passive and submissive. He is not necessarily defined by other S&Mers, nor does he have to define himself, as unmasculine because he happens to prefer the "bottom" role. A number of writers in the present book note that this is true (e.g., Weinberg, 1978; Kamel, 1980) and attempt theoretically to account for it.

Studying S&M as a social behavior enables us to probe the nature of a number of other phenomena. Gebhard pointed out that fantasy is extremely important to sadomasochistic encounters. "The average sadomasochistic session is usually scripted," he wrote, "the masochist must allegedly have done something meriting punishment, there must be threats and suspense before the punishment is meted out, etc. Often the phenomenon reminds one of a planned ritual or theatrical production" (Gebhard, 1969: 78). Looking at S&M scenes may, for example, give us some insight into how fantasies are produced and shared, the nature of the relationship between fantasy and sexuality, and the connection between play and sexual behavior.

The S&M world is a secret world. It has been described as a "velvet underground." Andreas Spengler (1977) noted that secrecy is one of the special norms of sadomasochists. Thus, a study of such behavior may help to reveal the nature of secrecy as a social phenomenon. The conditions under which secrets are developed, shared, kept, and revealed, and the functions of secrecy for social groups are important topics. We do know that different S&M worlds vary in the importance of secrecy to their participants and in the degree to which, and in the conditions under which, they make themselves visible. The gay "leathersex" subculture is much more visible than the heterosexual S&M world. Most large cities have gay S&M bars; with few exceptions, the contacts of heterosexual S&Mers are limited to private, small networks. The question is, why should this be the case? Are stigmatized groups such as homosexuals more tolerant of other sorts of unconventional sexual behavior? Is it that gays who are already "out" have (or feel that they have) less to lose by revealing sadomasochistic needs than do heterosexuals? Or is the explanation for the greater visibility of gay S&M that it occurs within an already existing structure and is therefore an easily accepted variation on a theme? Contacts among gay S&Mers seem to be more easily made in part because there are many more non-S&M settings in which people can find partners who may be willing to try an S&M scene as an extension of sex play.

Much sadomasochistic activity occurs in dyads and triads. Thus, studying S&M is likely to add to our knowledge of the ways in which small groups operate. How, for example, are decisions reached? How do people place limits on their behavior and that of others? What happens when these norms are violated? What is the connection between small S&M groups and the larger S&M world? How do people discover this world, get integrated into it, and develop contacts with potential partners? How do their identities, motives, and behavior develop and change over time? These and many other questions are answered by the articles that we have collected in this volume.

Finally, one good reason for studying sadomasochistic behavior is that it may be more prevalent in the larger society than one might suspect. Writers like Judith Coburn claim that there is a growing "S&M chic" in this country.

Sadomasochistic themes appear more and more in advertising, books, and movies. Adult sex toy shops and boutiques are becoming more and more prevalent. Even in 1969, Gebhard noted that

> The prevalence of unconscious sadomasochism is impossible to ascertain, but it must be large if one can make inferences from book and magazine sales and from box office reports. We do know that consciously recognized sexual arousal from sadomasochistic stimuli are not rare. The Institute for Sex Research found that one in eight females and one in five males were aroused by sadomasochistic stories. . . (p. 79).

All of the articles in this collection focus on sadomasochism as a form of social behavior. This means that these studies concern themselves with the interaction *between* individuals situated within a subcultural context. While they examine sadomasochism from a variety of viewpoints, all of the writers share some basic assumptions about S&M behavior. Without losing sight of the individual as participant, they are all concerned with the production and dissemination of social meanings as a central part of the sadomasochistic world. Their essays refrain from making the kinds of moral judgments often contaminating the work of earlier scholars.

In one way or another, each of the contributions to this book addresses the issues first outlined in the Gebhard article. They have been organized into three sections reflecting specific levels of analysis. The first section, "Selves," is concerned with the individual within the S&M milieu. The second section, "Scenes," focuses primarily upon the subcultural aspects of S&M. The third section, "Structures," discusses the organizational features of the sadomasochistic experience.

REFERENCES

Caprio, Frank S. *Variations in Sexual Behavior*. New York: Grove, 1955.

Coburn, Judith. "S&M," *New Times* 8 (Feb. 4): 43–50, 1977.

Ellis, Havelock. *Studies in the Psychology of Sex* (Vol. 1, Part 2), New York: Random House, 1942.

Freud, Sigmund. *The Basic Writings of Sigmund Freud* (A. A. Brill, trans. and ed.), New York: Modern Library, 1938.

Gebhard, Paul H. "Fetishism and Sadomasochism," pp. 71–80 in Jules H. Masserman, ed., *Dynamics of Deviant Sexuality*, New York: Grune & Stratton, 1969.

Kamel, G. W. Levi. "Leathersex: Meaningful Aspects of Gay Sadomasochism," *Deviant Behavior* 1: 171-191, 1980.

Krafft-Ebing, R. von. *Psychopathia Sexualis* (Franklin S. Klaf, trans.), New York: Stein and Day, 1965.

Lee, John Alan. "The Social Organization of Sexual Risk," *Alternative Lifestyles* 2 (Feb.): 69–100, 1979.

Mass, Lawrence. "Coming to Grips with Sadomasochism," *The Advocate* (April 5): 18–22, 1979.

Smith, Howard and Cathy Cox. "Scenes: Dialogue with a Dominatrix," *Village Voice* 24 (Jan. 29): 19–20, 1979.

Spengler, Andreas. "Manifest Sadomasochism of Males: Results of an Empirical Study," *Archives of Sexual Behavior* 6: 441–456, 1977.

Stekel, Wilhelm. *Sadism and Masochism,* New York: Grove Press, 1965.

Weinberg, Thomas S. "Sadism and Masochism: Sociological Perspectives," *Bulletin of the American Academy of Psychiatry and the Law* 6: 284–295, 1978.

Weinberg, Thomas S., and Gerhard Falk. "The Social Organization of Sadism and Masochism," *Deviant Behavior,* 1: 379–393, 1980.

Richard von Krafft-Ebing

Psychopathia Sexualis

Sadism: Association of Active Cruelty and Violence with Lust

Sadism, especially in its rudimentary manifestations, seems to be of common occurrence in the domain of sexual perversion. Sadism is the experience of sexual [sic] pleasurable sensations (including orgasm) produced by acts of cruelty, bodily punishment afflicted on one's own person or when witnessed in others, be they animals or human beings. It may also consist of an innate desire to humiliate, hurt, wound or even destroy others in order thereby to create sexual pleasure in one's self.

Thus it will happen that one of the consorts in sexual heat will strike, bite or pinch the other, that kissing degenerates into biting. Lovers and young married couples are fond of teasing each other, they wrestle together "just for fun," indulge in all sorts of horseplay. The transition from these atavistic manifestations, which no doubt belong to the sphere of physiological sexuality, to the most monstrous acts of destruction of the consort's life can be readily traced.

Where the husband forces the wife by menaces and other violent means to the conjugal act, we can no longer describe such as a normal physiological manifestation, but must ascribe it to sadistic impulses. It seems probable that this sadistic force is developed by the natural shyness and modesty of women towards the aggressive manners of the male, especially during the earlier periods of married life and particularly where the husband is hypersexual. Woman no doubt derives pleasure from her innate coyness and the final victory of man affords her intense and refined gratification. Hence the frequent recurrence of these little love comedies. . . .

In the civilized man of today, in so far as he is untainted, associations between lust and cruelty are found, but in a weak and rather rudimentary degree. If such therefore occur and in fact even light atrocious manifestations thereof, they must be attributed to distorted dispositions (sexual and motoric spheres).

They are due to an awakening of latent psychical dispositions, occasioned by external circumstances which in no way affect the normal individual. They are not accidental deviations of sentiment or instinct in the sense as given by the modern doctrine of association. Sadistic sensations may often be traced back to early childhood and exist during a period of life when their revival can by no manner of means be attributed to external impressions, much less to sexual temper.

Sadism must, therefore, like Masochism and the antipathic sexual instinct, be counted among the primitive anomalies of the sexual life. It is a disturbance (a deviation) in the evolution of psychosexual processes sprouting from the soil of psychical degeneration.

That lust and cruelty often occur together is a fact that has long been recognized and is frequently observed. Writers of all kinds have called attention to this phenomenon. . . .

In an attempt to explain the association of lust and cruelty, it is necessary to return to a consideration of the quasi-physiological cases, in which, at the moment of most intense lust, very excitable individuals, who are otherwise normal, commit such acts as biting and scratching, which are usually due to anger. It must further be remembered that love and anger are not only the most intense emotions, but also the only two forms of robust emotion. Both seek their object, try to possess themselves of it, and naturally exhaust themselves in a physical effect on it; both throw the psycho-motor sphere into the most intense excitement, and thus, by means of this excitation, reach their normal expression.

From this standpoint it is clear how lust impels to acts that otherwise are expressive of anger. The one, like the other, is a state of exaltation, an intense excitation of the entire psycho-motor sphere. Thus there arises an impulse to react on the object that induces the stimulus, in every possible way, and with the greatest intensity. Just as maniacal exaltation easily passes to raging destructiveness, so exaltation of the sexual emotion often induces an impulse to spend itself in senseless and apparently harmful acts. To a certain extent these are psychical accompaniments; but it is not simply an unconscious excitation of innervation of muscles (which also sometimes occurs as blind violence); it is a true hyperbole, a desire to exert the utmost possible effect upon the individual giving rise to the stimulus. The most intense means, however, is the infliction of pain.

Through such cases of infliction of pain during the most intense emotion of lust, we approach the cases in which a real injury, wound, or death is inflicted on the victim. In these cases the impulse to cruelty which may accompany the emotion of lust, becomes unbounded in a psychopathic individual; and, at the same time, owing to defect of moral feeling, all normal inhibitory ideas are absent or weakened.

Such monstrous, sadistic acts have, however, in men, in whom they are much more frequent than in women, another source in physiological conditions. In the intercourse of the sexes, the active or aggressive role belongs to man; woman remains passive, defensive. It affords man great pleasure to win a woman, to conquer her; and in the art of love making, the modesty of woman, who keeps herself on the defensive until the moment of surrender, is an element of great psychological significance and importance. Under normal conditions man meets obstacles which it is his part to overcome, and for which nature has given him an aggressive character. This aggressive character, however, under pathological conditions may likewise be excessively developed, and express itself in an impulse to subdue absolutely the object of desire, even to destroy or kill it.

If both these constituent elements occur together—the abnormally intensified impulse to a violent reaction towards the object of the stimulus, and the abnormally intensified desire to conquer the woman—then the most violent outbreaks of sadism occur.

Sadism is thus nothing else than an excessive and monstrous pathological intensification of phenomena—possible, too, in normal conditions in rudimental forms—which accompany the psychical sexual life, particularly in males. It is of course not at all necessary, and not even the rule, that the sadistic individual should be conscious of his instinct. What he feels is, as a rule, only the impulse to cruel and violent treatment of the opposite sex, and the coloring of the idea of such acts with lustful feelings. Thus arises a powerful impulse to commit the imagined deeds. In as far as the actual motives of this instinct are not comprehended by the individual, the sadistic acts have the character of impulsive deeds.

When the association of lust and cruelty is present, not only does the lustful emotion awaken the impulse to cruelty, but *vice versa*; cruel ideas and acts of cruelty cause sexual excitement, and in this way are used by perverse individuals.

MASOCHISM: THE ASSOCIATION OF PASSIVELY ENDURED CRUELTY
AND VIOLENCE WITH LUST

Masochism is the opposite of sadism. While the latter is the desire to cause pain and use force, the former is the wish to suffer pain and be subjected to force.

By masochism I understand a peculiar perversion of the psychical sexual life in which the individual affected, in sexual feeling and thought, is controlled by the idea of being completely and unconditionally subject to the will of a person of the opposite sex; of being treated by this person as by a master, humiliated and abused. This idea is colored by lustful feeling; the masochist lives in fantasies, in which he creates situations of this kind and often attempts to realize them. By this perversion his sexual instinct is often made more or less insensible to the normal charms of the opposite sex — incapable of a normal sexual life — psychically impotent. But this psychical impotence does not in any way depend upon a horror of the opposite sex, but upon the fact that the perverse instinct finds an adequate satisfaction differing from the normal — in woman, to be sure, but not in coitus.

But cases also occur in which with the perverse impulse there is still some sensibility to normal stimuli, and intercourse under normal conditions takes place. In other cases the impotence is not purely psychical, but physical, *i.e.,* spinal; for this perversion, like almost all other perversions of the sexual instinct, is developed only on the basis of a psychopathic and, for the most part, hereditarily tainted individuality; and as a rule such individuals are given to excesses, particularly masturbation, to which the difficulty of attaining what their fancy creates drives them again and again.

I feel justified in calling this sexual anomaly "Masochism," because the author *Sacher-Masoch* frequently made this perversion, which up to his time was quite unknown to the scientific world as such, the substratum of his writings. I followed thereby the scientific formation of the term "Daltonism," from *Dalton,* the discoverer of color-blindness.

During recent years facts have been advanced which prove that Sacher-Masoch was not only the poet of Masochism, but that he himself was afflicted with this anomaly. Although these proofs were communicated to me without restriction, I refrain from giving them to the public. I refute the accusation that I have coupled the name of a revered author with a perversion of the sexual instinct, which has been made against me by some admirers of the author and by some critics of my book. As a man Sacher-Masoch cannot lose anything in the estimation of his cultured fellow-beings simply because he was afflicted with an anomaly of his sexual feelings. As an author he suffered severe injury so far as the influence and intrinsic merit of his work is concerned, for so long and whenever he eliminated his perversion from his literary efforts, he was a gifted writer, and as such would have achieved real greatness had he been actuated by normally sexual feelings. In this respect he is a remarkable example of the powerful influence exercised by the sexual life — be it in the good or evil sense — over the formation and direction of man's mind.

The number of cases of undoubted masochism thus far observed is very large. Whether masochism occurs associated with normal sexual instincts, or exclusively controls the individual; whether or not, and to what extent, the individual subject to this perversion strives to realize his peculiar fancies;

whether or not, he has thus more or less diminished his virility—depends upon the degree of intensity of the perversion in the single case, upon the strength of the opposing ethical and aesthetic motives, and the relative power of the physical and mental organization of the affected individual. From the psychopathic point of view, the essential and common element in all these cases is *the fact that the sexual instinct is directed to ideas of subjugation and abuse by the opposite sex.*

Whatever has been said with reference to the impulsive character (indistinctness of motive) of the resulting acts and with reference to the original (congenital) nature of the perversion in sadism, is also true in masochism.

In masochism there is a gradation of the acts from the most repulsive and monstrous to the silliest, regulated by the degree of intensity of the perverse instinct and the power of the remnants of moral and aesthetic countermotives. The extreme consequences of masochism, however, are checked by the instinct of self-preservation, and therefore murder and serious injury, which may be committed in sadistic excitement, have here in reality, so far as known, no passive equivalent. But the perverse desires of masochistic individuals may in imagination attain these extreme consequences.

Moreover, the acts to which masochists resort are in some cases performed in connection with coitus, *i.e.,* as preparatory measures; in others, as substitutes for coitus when this is impossible. This, too, depends only upon the condition of sexual power, which has been diminished for the most part physically and mentally by the activity of the sexual ideas in the perverse direction, and not upon the nature of the act itself.

Sigmund Freud

Sadism and Masochism

The tendency to cause pain to the sexual object and its opposite, the most frequent and most significant of all perversions, was designated in its two forms by Krafft-Ebing as sadism for the active form, and masochism for the passive form. Other authors prefer the narrower term, *algolagnia,* which emphasizes the pleasure in pain and cruelty, whereas the terms selected by Krafft-Ebing place the pleasure secured in all kinds of humility and submission in the foreground.

The roots of active algolagnia, sadism, can be readily demonstrable in the normal individual. The sexuality of most men shows an admixture of aggression, of a desire to subdue, the biological significance of which lies in the necessity for overcoming the resistance of the sexual object by actions other than mere *courting.* Sadism would then correspond to an aggressive component of the sexual instinct which has become independent and exaggerated and has been brought to the foreground by displacement.

The concept of sadism fluctuates in everyday speech from a mere active or impetuous attitude towards the sexual object to an absolute attachment of the gratification to the subjection and maltreatment of the object. Strictly speaking, only the last extreme case can claim the name of perversion.

Similarly, the designation masochism comprises all passive attitudes to the sexual life and to the sexual object: in its most extreme form the gratification is connected with suffering of physical or mental pain at the hands of the sexual object. Masochism as a perversion seems further removed from the normal sexual goal than its opposite. It may even be doubted whether it

Excerpted from Sigmund Freud, *The Basic Writings of Sigmund Freud* (A. A. Brill, trans. and ed.) New York: The Modern Library, 1938, pp. 569-571.

ever is primary and whether it does not more often originate through transformation from sadism.[1] It can often be recognized that masochism is nothing but a continuation of sadism directed against one's own person in which the latter at first takes the place of the sexual object. Clinical analysis of extreme cases of masochistic perversions show that there is a cooperation of a large series of factors which exaggerate and fix the original passive sexual attitude (castration complex, guilt).

The pain which is here overcome ranks with the loathing and shame which are the resistances opposed to the libido.

Sadism and masochism occupy a special place in the perversions, for the contrast of activity and passivity lying at their bases belong to the common traits of the sexual life.

That cruelty and the sexual instinct are most intimately connected is beyond doubt taught by the history of civilization, but in the explanation of this connection no one has gone beyond the accentuation of the aggressive factors of the libido. The aggression which is mixed with the sexual instinct is, according to some authors, a remnant of cannibalistic lust — that is, a participation of the domination apparatus, which serves also for the gratification of the other ontogenetically older great need.[2] It has also been claimed that every pain contains in itself the possibility of a pleasurable sensation. Let us be satisfied with the impression that the explanation given concerning this perversion is by no means satisfactory and that it is possible that many psychic strivings unite herein into one effect.[3]

The most striking peculiarity of this perversion lies in the fact that its active and passive forms are regularly encountered together in the same person. He who experiences pleasure by causing pain to others in sexual relations is also capable of experiencing pain in sexual relations as pleasure. A sadist is simultaneously a masochist, though either the active or the passive side of the perversion may be more strongly developed in him and thus, represent his preponderant sexual activity.[4]

We, thus, see that certain perverted tendencies regularly appear in contrasting pairs, which . . . is of great theoretical value. It is furthermore clear that the existence of the contrast, sadism and masochism, can not readily be attributed to the mixture of aggression. On the other hand, one may be tempted to connect each synchronously existing contrast with the united contrast of male and female in bi-sexuality, the significance of which is reduced in psychoanalysis to the contrast of activity and passivity.

NOTES

1. Later reflections which can be supported by definite evidence concerning the structure of the mental systems and of the activities of instincts therein, have changed my judgment concerning masochism very widely,

I have been led to recognize a primary erotogenic masochism from which there develops two later forms, a feminine and a moral masochism. Through a turning back of an unconsumed sadism directed against one-self during life there arises a secondary masochism which is added to the primary masochism. (See Freud, Das ökonomische Problem des Maso-chisten, Int. Zeit. f. Psa, 10, 121, 1924. Translated into English in *Collected Papers,* Vol. 2, p. 255. Hogarth Press.)

2. Cf. here the later studies on the pregenital phases of the sexual develop-ment, in which this view is confirmed.
3. From the researches just cited, the contrasted pair, sadism-masochism, originates from a special source of impulses and is to be differentiated from the other "perversions."
4. Instead of substantiating this statement by many examples, I will merely cite Havelock Ellis (*The Sexual Impulse,* 1903): "All known cases of sadism and masochism even those cited by Krafft-Ebing always show (as has already been shown by Colin, Scott, and Fere) traces of both groups of manifestations in the same individual."

Havelock Ellis

Studies in the Psychology of Sex

In the foregoing rapid survey of the great group of manifestations in which
the sexual emotions come into intimate relationship with pain, it has become
fairly clear that the ordinary division between "sadism" and "masochism,"
convenient as these terms may be, had a very slight correspondence with
facts. Sadism and masochism may be regarded as complementary emotional
states; they cannot be regarded as opposed states. Even de Sade himself, we
have seen, can scarcely be regarded as a pure sadist. A passage in one of his
works expressing regret that sadistic feeling is rare among women, as well as
his definite recognition of the fact that the suffering of pain may call forth
voluptuous emotions, shows that he was not insensitive to the charms of
masochistic experience, and it is evident that a merely bloodthirsty vampire,
sane or insane, could never have retained, as de Sade retained, the undying
devotion of two women so superior in heart and intelligence as his wife and
sister-in-law. . . . It is clear that, apart from the organically morbid twist
by which he obtained sexual satisfaction in his partner's pain—a craving
which was, for the most part, only gratified in imaginary visions developed
to an inhuman extent under the influence of solitude—de Sade was simply
to those who knew him, *"un aimable mauvais sujet"* gifted with exceptional
intellectual powers. Unless we realize this we run the risk of confounding
de Sade and his like with men of whom Judge Jeffreys was the sinister type.

Excerpted from Havelock Ellis, *Studies in the Pathology of Sex,* Volume III, *Analysis of the
Sexual Impulse, Love and Pain, The Sexual Impulse in Women,* Second Edition, Revised and
Enlarged, Philadelphia: F. A. Davis Company, 1926: pp. 159-160, 166, 171-172, 175-176. This
1926 version of Ellis's work is a reissue of the 1913 revised and expanded second edition. The
first edition was originally published in 1903. Reprinted by permission of Professor Francois
Lafitte, trustee of the Havelock Ellis Estate.

It is necessary to emphasize this point because there can be no doubt that de Sade is really a typical instance of the group of perversions he represents, and when we understand that it is pain only, and not cruelty, that is the essential in this group of manifestations we begin to come nearer to their explanation. The masochist desires to experience pain, but he generally desires that it should be inflicted in love; the sadist desires to inflict pain, but in some cases, if not in most, he desires that it should be felt as love. How far de Sade consciously desired that the pain he sought to inflict should be felt as pleasure it may not now be possible to discover, except by indirect inference, but the confessions of sadists show that such a desire is quite commonly essential. . . .

We have thus to recognize that sadism by no means involves any love of inflicting pain outside the sphere of sexual emotion, and is even compatible with a high degree of general tender-heartedness. We have also to recognize that even within the sexual sphere the sadist by no means wishes to exclude the victim's pleasure, and may even regard that pleasure as essential to his own satisfaction. We have, further, to recognize that, in view of the close connection between sadism and masochism, it is highly probable that in some cases the sadist is really a disguised masochist and enjoys his victim's pain because he identifies himself with that pain.

But there is a further group of cases, and a very important group, on account of the light it throws on the essential nature of these phenomena, and that is the group in which the thought or the spectacle of pain acts as a sexual stimulant, without the subject identifying himself clearly either with the inflicter or the sufferer of the pain. Such cases are sometimes classed as sadistic; but this is incorrect, for they might just as truly be called masochistic. The term algolagnia might properly be applied to them (and Eulenburg now classes them as "ideal algolagnia"), for they reveal an undifferentiated connection between sexual excitement and pain not developed into either active or passive participation. Such feelings may arise sporadically in persons in whom no sadistic or masochistic perversion can be said to exist, though they usually appear in individuals of neurotic temperament. . . .

We have seen that the distinction between "sadism" and "masochism" cannot be maintained; not only was even de Sade himself something of a masochist and Sacher-Masoch something of a sadist, but between these two extreme groups of phenomena there is a central group in which the algolagnia is neither active nor passive. "Sadism" and "masochism" are simply convenient clinical terms for classes of manifestations which quite commonly occur in the same person. We have further found that — as might have been anticipated in view of the foregoing result — it is scarcely correct to use the word "cruelty" in connection with the phenomena we have been considering. The persons who experience these impulses usually show no love of cruelty outside the sphere of sexual emotion; they may even be very intolerant of cruelty. Even when their sexual impulses come into play they may still desire to secure the pleasure of the persons who arouse their sexual emotions, even though it may not be often true that those who desire to inflict pain at these moments identify themselves with the feelings of those on whom they inflict it. We have thus seen that when we take a comprehensive survey of all these phenomena a somewhat general formula will alone cover them. Our conclusion so far must be that under certain abnormal circumstances pain, more especially the mental representation of pain, acts as a powerful sexual stimulant.

The reader, however, who has followed the discussion to this point will be prepared to take the next and final step in our discussion and to reach a more definite conclusion. The question naturally arises: by what process does pain or its mental representation thus act as a sexual stimulant? The answer has over and over again been suggested by the facts brought forward in this study. Pain acts as a sexual stimulant because it is the most powerful of all methods for arousing emotion. . . .

In the ordinary healthy organism, however, although the stimulants of strong emotion may be vaguely pleasurable, they do not have more than a general action on the sexual sphere, nor are they required for the due action of the sexual mechanism. But in a slightly abnormal organism — whether the anomaly is due to a congenital neuropathic condition, or to a possibly acquired neurasthenic condition, or merely to the physiological inadequacy of childhood or old age — the balance of nervous energy is less favorable for the adequate play of the ordinary energies in courtship. The sexual impulse is itself usually weaker, even when, as often happens, its irritability assumes the fallacious appearance of strength. It has become unusually sensitive to unusual stimuli and also, it is possible — perhaps as a result of those conditions — more liable to atavistic manifestations. An organism in this state becomes peculiarly apt to seize on the automatic sources of energy generated by emotion. The parched sexual instinct greedily drinks up and absorbs the force it obtains by applying abnormal stimuli to its emotional apparatus. It becomes largely, if not solely, dependent on the energy thus secured. The abnormal organism in this respect may become as dependent on anger or fear, and for the same reason, as in other respects it may become dependent on alcohol.

Paul H. Gebhard

Sadomasochism

Sadomasochism may be operationally defined as obtaining sexual arousal through receiving or giving physical or mental pain. Unlike fetishism, analogues are common among other mammalian species wherein coitus is preceded by behavior which under other circumstances would be interpreted as combative. Temporary phases of actual fighting may be interspread in such pre-coital activity. In some species, such as mink, sexual activity not infrequently results in considerable wounds. This pre-coital activity has definite neurophysiological value in establishing, or reinforcing, many of the physiological concomitants of sexual arousal such as increased pulse and blood pressure, hyperventilation, and muscular tension. Indeed one may elicit sexual behavior in some animals by exciting them with non-sexual stimuli. This may explain why sadomasochism is used as a crutch by aging men in our society who require some extra impetus to achieve arousal. From a phylogenetic viewpoint it is no surprise to find sadomasochism in human beings.

Sadomasochism is embedded in our culture since our culture operates on the basis of dominance-submission relationships, and aggression is socially valued. Even our gender relationships have been formulated in a framework conducive to sadomasochism: the male is supposed to be dominant and aggressive sexually and the female reluctant or submissive. Violence and sex are commingled to make a profitable package to sell through the mass media. This is no innovation—for centuries the masochistic damsel in distress has been victimized by the evil sadist who is finally defeated by the hero through violent means.

Excerpted from Paul H. Gebhard, "Fetishism and Sadomasochism," pp. 71-80 in Jules Masserman, M.D., ed. *Dynamics of Deviant Sexuality: Scientific Proceedings of the American Academy of Psychoanalysis,* New York: Grune & Stratton, 1969, pp. 77-80. Reprinted by permission of Grune & Stratton and the Kinsey Institute for Research in Sex, Gender & Reproduction, Inc., as well as the author.

Relatively few sadomasochists are exclusively sadists or exclusively masochists; there is generally a mixture with one aspect predominant. This mixing is sometimes necessitated by circumstances: sexual partners are extremely difficult to find and consequently, for example, if two masochists meet they are obliged to take turns at the sadist role. This role-taking is made easier by ability to project. The masochist playing the sadist may fantasy himself receiving the pain he is inflicting.

Sadists are far rarer than masochists, and female sadists are so highly prized that masochists will travel hundreds of miles to meet them. I postulate that this imbalance between sadists and masochists is a product of our culture wherein physical violence, particularly to someone of the opposite gender, is taboo and productive of intense guilt. To strike is sin; to be struck is guiltless or even virtuous in a martyrdom sense. Even more psychodynamically important is masochism as an expiation for the sin of sexuality. During childhood, puberty, and part of adolescence sexual behavior is punished and it is easy to form an association between sexual pleasure and punishment. The masochist has a nice guilt relieving system — he gets his punishment simultaneously with his sexual pleasure or else is entitled to his pleasure by first enduring the punishment.

It is important to realize that pain *per se* is not attractive to the masochist, and generally not to the sadist, unless it occurs in an arranged situation. Accidental pain is not perceived as pleasurable or sexual. The average sadomasochistic session is usually scripted: the masochist must allegedly have done something meriting punishment, there must be threats and suspense before the punishment is meted out, etc. Often the phenomenon reminds one of a planned ritual or theatrical production. Indeed, sado-masochistic prostitutes often report their clients give them specialized instructions to follow. Genet's *Balcony* is true to life. When one appreciates this one realizes that often in the relationship the sadist is not truly in charge — the sadist is merely servicing the masochist. The sadist must develop an extraordinary perceptiveness to know when to continue, despite cries and protests, and when to cease. A sadist who goes too far or stops prematurely may find his ineptitude has cost him a sexual partner. Not infrequently sadomasochistic activity is interspersed with loving and tender-ness. This alternation makes the process far more powerful. Police and brainwashers use the same technique of alternate brutality and sympathy to break their subjects.

Sadomasochism is extremely complex. Some achieve orgasm during the pain; in other cases the sadomasochism only constitutes the foreplay and the session culminates in conventional sexual behavior. Some masochists dislike the pain while it is being inflicted, but obtain gratification by anticipation of the pain or by thinking about it after it has ceased. Lastly, there are the bondage people who do not enjoy pain but are stimulated by constraint, mild discomfort, and a sense of helplessness. Bondage has both sadistic and masochistic aspects. The sadist has the pleasure of rendering his partner helpless and at his mercy—a favorite sexual theme in mythology, literature, and fantasy. The masochist bondage enthusiast enjoys not only the restraint itself but the guilt relieving knowledge that if anything sexual occurs it is not his or her fault. Also as Dr. Douglas Alcorn points out, some persons derive a sense of comfort and security from physical constraint. Lastly, the hood, often used in bondage, offers the advantage of depersonalization and heightens the helplessness through interfering with sight, hearing and vocalization.

Both sadomasochism and bondage are often replete with fetish items including specialized clothing and restraint or torture devices. All this offers the devotee substantial additional gratification. The average heterosexual or homosexual has relatively little paraphernalia for supplementary pleasure and it offers scant opportunity for ingenuity or creativity.

The prevalence of unconscious sadomasochism is impossible to ascertain, but it must be large if one can make inferences from book and magazine sales and from box office reports. We do know that consciously recognized sexual arousal from sadomasochistic stimuli are not rare. The Institute for Sex Research found that about one in eight females and one in five males were aroused by sadomasochistic stories, and roughly half of both sexes were aroused by being bitten.

The etiology of sadomasochism, while the subject of much writing especially in the form of interminable German books, is not well understood. In individual cases the genesis may be clear as psychoanalysis and psychiatry amply demonstrates, but these individualistic explanations do not suffice for the phenomenon as a whole. After all, the supply of English headmasters and Austrian girl friends is limited. We must turn to broad hypotheses, and I will offer a rather simplistic one.

First, we may assume on the basis of mammalian studies and history that we humans have built-in aggressive tendencies. Second, it is equally clear that males are on the whole more aggressive than females. Experiments indicate this is in large part an endocrine matter: androgens elicit or enhance aggression. Thirdly, animal and human social organization is generally based on a dominance-submissiveness relationship, a peck-order. Fourthly, when one couples the difficulties of sexual gratification with the problems involved in living in a peck-order society, one has an endless source of frustration which lends itself to expression in pathological combinations of sex and violence. Note that in our own culture when we wish to say that someone was badly victimized we use sexual terms such as, "he got screwed." From a rational viewpoint we should apply the words "he got screwed" to someone who had had a pleasurable experience, but we have unfortunately mixed sex with dominance-submissiveness behavior.

This using sex as a symbol brings up the puzzle as to why explicitly sexual sadomasochism, like fetishism, seems the monopoly of well-developed civilizations. One never hears of an aged Polynesian having to be flogged to obtain an erection, and for all their torture and bloodshed there seem to have been no De Sades amongst the Plains Indians or Aztecs. While it is true that in various preliterate societies sexual activity often involves moderate scratching and biting, well-developed sadomasochism as a life-style is conspicuous by its absence. It may be that a society must be extremely complex and heavily reliant upon symbolism before the inescapable repressions and frustrations of life in such a society can be expressed symbolically in sadomasochism. Sadomasochism is beautifully suited to symbolism: what better proof of power and status is there than inflicting humiliation or pain upon someone who does not retaliate? And what better proof of love is there than enduring or even seeking such treatment?

REFERENCE

Alcorn, Douglass: Personal communication.

SELVES
S&M IDENTITIES

Introduction

In the first essay, "Coming to Grips with Sadomasochism," Lawrence Mass, a physician, discusses the present state of scientific ignorance about S&M and suggests that the psychiatric viewpoints dominating the field have been too narrow, too individualistic, and too moralistic. In short, Mass outlines both lay and scientific attempts at "coming to grips with sadomasochism." Largely a critique of both Puritanism and psychoanalysis, Mass's essay helps to identify a series of fascinating questions about S&M that the authors who follow will attempt to develop further.

In the most comprehensive research project contained in this collection, Andreas Spengler's "Manifest Sadomasochism of Males: Results of an Empirical Study" combines both quantitative and qualitative data to link identity formation with the subculture of sadomasochism. A similar linkage is at least implicit in Paul Gebhard's early statement, since he posits a relationship between individual expressions of sadomasochism and the frustrations of civilized social life. Spengler draws several careful conclusions about sexual practices such as the uses of S&M equipment, masturbation, and dominance-submission techniques, as well as examining sexual preferences such as role alternatives, erotic fantasies and wishes, and sexual orientation. Aspects of the S&M identity including coming-out processes, self-perception, and self-acceptance are extensively explored.

G. W. Levi Kamel's "The Leather Career: On Becoming a Sadomasochist" describes in detail the stages in identity formation for gay male sadomasochists, one of the three groups surveyed by Dr. Spengler. Kamel examines the acquisition of a "leatherman" identity as a dynamic process involving attempts at "sense-making" on the part of men entering the S&M world. Kamel illustrates the interplay between what one observes and how one interprets and applies this information.

43

The essay entitled "Dialogue with a Dominatrix" by Howard Smith and Cathy Cox is important because of its implications for identity formation and management of self within a deviant social context. In it "Mistress Rose," a prostitute and professional dominatrix with many male clients, provides us with some of the rich detail of heterosexual S&M, while suggesting the complexity of the relationship between the individual participant and the S&M scene.

The last selection, "Autobiography of a Dominatrix," is included to provide a contrast to the socialization of Mistress Rose. Unlike Rose, Juliette follows an uncharted path into S&M. Rather than learning S&M through imitation, as Mistress Rose did in learning from her mother, Juliette learns through "sense-making," redefining as desirable each step of the way into S&M. In further contrast, S&M served as an end in itself for Mistress Rose; her role as a prostitute appears to be less important to her than her role as a dominatrix. Being a dominatrix was not just a job to Mistress Rose; her identity was only secondarily that of a prostitute. Juliette, however, sees S&M as a means to an end, that of making a living. Juliette identifies herself primarily as a prostitute. Thus, she reports having been amazed when she met a woman who, like Mistress Rose, was involved in S&M "on her own time."

Lawrence Mass

Coming to Grips with Sadomasochism

The sexual revolution has seen battle on every major front of human sexual behavior, except one. The province of sadomasochism remains unclaimed and largely unchallenged by sex researchers, sociobiologists, medical psychologists, biological psychiatrists—in short, by any of the younger disciplines currently involved in the study of human sexuality. By default, sadomasochism remains the imperative territory of psychoanalytic psychiatry.

In an earlier *Advocate* piece, "Shackles and Guilt" (Issue 234), Mark Thompson explores the unhappiness of sexuality suppressed by cultural shackles. The author indicates that sadomasochists are among several sexual minorities designated or characterized as deviant by social, religious or political institutions. Thompson expresses sympathy for those who seek legitimization of their right to the private, consensual pursuit of sexual pleasure.

The future liberalization of laws would seem to be an appropriate outcome of the ongoing liberalization of attitudes toward sexual conduct. But can "sadomasochism" be part of "mature" or "normal" sexuality? Can increasing tolerance render it more so?

The subject of sadomasochism should be of special concern to homosexuals. From outside the gay community, religious and political oppression has traditionally focused on the "unnatural," "perverse" and "violent" nature of homosexual acts. "Effeminate self-abusers" is what Anita Bryant calls homosexuals. As she explains in her interview with *Playboy* (5/1979):

A revised version of an article that originally appeared in *The Advocate*, (April 5, 1979): pp. 18–22. Copyright © 1979 by Lawrence Mass.

"The homosexual act is just the beginning of the depravity. It then leads to—what's the word?—sadomasochism."

Within the gay community, these attacks are not defused by the increasing visibility of the "leather" subculture. Bars, baths, magazines, "toy" stores and private clubs catering to sadomasochistic tastes have proliferated, alongside the more respectable artifacts of a community in the throes of "coming out." *Vogue* models in black leather notwithstanding, sadomasochistic behavior among heterosexuals is less overtly subcultural and is contrastingly less conspicuous.

In fact, many individuals of both genders and of a range of sexual preferences are expressing interest in the phenomenon of overt sexual sadomasochism. Those for whom the experience is consciously foreign fear that S&M may indeed be unnatural, perverse, and violent. Others, especially those who identify themselves as sadomasochists, defend their deviation as a healthy, consensual recognition and ritualization of otherwise repressed impulses, otherwise expressed nonsexually as destructive aggression or its obverse, moral masochism. Some think it's no more than a fashion, a marketable emphasis on violence entirely consistent with hedonistic trends in the culture at large.

The diversity of questions about sadomasochism seems to have generated surprisingly little in the way of hard core scientific data. Major obstacles to its study are predictable. The greatest, of course, is that of social taboo. Few researchers and fewer funding resources are willing to risk the vulnerabilities in a subject so controversial, so abhorrent to the conscious standards of morality.

In the introduction to their provocative study *S-M: The Last Taboo* (1974), psychologists Gerald and Caroline Greene comment on this paucity of reliable scientific information:

> We are a 'scientific' culture, given to attaching electrodes to nipple and navel and thereby hoping to verify something called sexual response. To date, however, there has been no equivalent investigation into S-M, nor could any such seem anything but remotely possible.

Paul Gebhard, acting director of the (Kinsey) Institute for Sex Research, emphasizes the ubiquity of this deviation (as did Freud):

> These quantitative aspects fully justify fetishism and sadomasochism receiving more attention. . . in our present state of knowledge, we cannot offer any seasoned theories buttressed by factual data. . . . Such studies will be difficult because most sadomasochists, unlike most homosexuals, are not striving for social tolerance and recognition. They prefer to remain mysteriously secret, considering themselves a hidden elite. (Mass, Lawrence, personal correspondence '79)

Not everyone would agree with Dr. Gebhard's conjecture. The Eulenspiegel Society of New York is the nation's largest organization of self-proclaimed sadomasochists. The Society's "Proclamation of Rights" includes the "right to publicize activities and views—freely, without fear of occupational or professional repercussion—thereby raising the consciousness of both the public and ourselves regarding sexual minorities and sexual freedoms."

As a population constituency, who *are* sadomasochists? What are their age, gender, sexual orientation, racial, geographic, and socioeconomic distributions? What are their levels of intelligence and psychological adjustment? Apart from their sexual behavior, do they differ by measurable parameters from so-called normal or average individuals?

The only completed empirical study of sadomasochists, in fact, has been conducted by sex researchers in Germany, rather than by psychiatrists in the United States. This is consistent with another cultural trend, one that has seen the credibility of opinion about human sexual behavior shift progressively from the temples of psychiatry to the laboratories of sex research.

The observation of this shift provides C. A. Tripp's *Homosexual Matrix* with much of its ammunition. Despite its emotional tone and sometimes frail documentation, his chapter on "The Question of Psychotherapy" pins its target. Tripp's bold contention that "a really major blow has been delivered to the whole field of psychotherapy from the thoroughgoing and quiet repudiation by scientists" is probably correct. His criticism here is primarily directed at the kind of psychoanalytic psychotherapy that treats homosexuality *per se* as pathology; the kind of therapy that in the fingertips of its leading contemporary exponent, Dr. Charles Socarides, tells but never shows the carrot-like cure that is dangled before the patient as his therapeutic goal: maturation to heterosexuality (the psychoanalytic pilgrimage from mommy to Menscheit). In the prestigious new Kinsey study, *Homosexualities,* and in the forthcoming Masters and Johnson study of homosexuality, these scientists may be dealing the *coup de grace* to all such cure-directed therapy. Doubtless these same scientsts will eventually gather and interpret many of the facts about sadomasochism, leaving the ilk of Dr. Socarides in the shrinking hemlines of this same, increasingly unbecoming, shift of credibility.

The inevitable border disputes between psychiatry and sex research could result in a truce. Despite orthodox extremes in one camp or the other, there may be enough mutual flexibility and complementarity for a state of peaceful coexistence. Then again, there may not be.

Even at their present tortoise-like pace, the sex researchers seem to be cautiously advancing toward the conclusion that overt sadomasochistic behavior may in some instances be a normal, not necessarily regressive, variance of healthy erotosexual expression. This parallels their work with homosexuals. In *Homosexualities,* principal authors Bell and Weinberg suggest that

> the least ambiguous finding in our investigation is that homosexuality is not necessarily related to pathology. . . . Moreover, it should be recognized that what has survival value in a heterosexual context may be destructive in a homosexual context, and vice versa. Life-enhancing mechanisms used by heterosexual men and women should not necessarily be used as the standard by which to judge the degree of homosexuals' adjustments.

This objectivity is also evident in the modest empirical study of sadomasochists eariler alluded to. In "Manifest Sadomasochism in Males: Results of an Empirical Study" (*Archives of Sexual Behavior,* 12/1977), A. Spengler concluded that

> direct or indirect integration into the deviant subculture makes possible the mitigation of conflicts arising from the deviant sexual orientation and the mitigation of poor acceptance of these desires. Only a minority of those studied appeared not to have found a way to positive self-acceptance.

The study quietly suggests that sadomasochism, however repellent to superficial cultural standards, is a form of consensual erotosexual bonding. Those individuals who have come to terms with their sexuality, as manifest by subcultural involvement, appear to be well adjusted.

Here in the United States, the only attempt at a scientific evaluation of sadomasochists is being conducted by sexologist Charles Moser under the auspices of San Francisco's Institute for the Advanced Study of Human Sexuality. Its academic dean is former Kinsey associate, Wardell Pomeroy. In a survey of 178 male and 47 female club-member sadomasochists, Moser administered the same 17-point psychological functioning inventory that Weinberg and Williams used in their study of male homosexuals. Though his work is ongoing, Moser maintains that sadomasochists are scoring somewhere between the male homosexuals of the Weinberg-Williams study and their heterosexual controls. The psychological adjustment of male sadomasochists, in other words, is similar to that of male homosexuals in our society. There is no evidence to suggest that it is significantly deficient.

Psychiatric viewpoints are generally less permissive and would suffer less criticism. New York psychotherapist and sociologist Susanne P. Schad-Somers has worked extensively with sadomasochistic couples, both homosexual and heterosexual. In her new book [1982], which will be devoted to the subject of reconciliation therapy with such couples, she presents her essentially analytic point of view. Not surprisingly, she believes that "sadomasochism is an adaptive response to the sadism of a parent. The price paid for maintaining the illusion of mother's love is *introjection* (psychic incorporation of the sadistic parent)." Challenging the tolerant inconclusiveness of the sex researchers, she counters that the establishment of a deviant subculture, with its undeniable secondary gains for the individual participant, does not necessarily legitimize the deviant behavior as moral, normal, or healthy. In the Greene study, the authors contend that S&M allows our aggressive instincts to be released in the bedroom rather than on the battlefield through bloodshed, violent crimes, or racism. But Dr. Schad-Somers is impatient with such reasoning. In a personal communication she told me, "That's just not the way it is." In other words, she feels that sadomasochism is not a part of mature sexuality.

In *A Sexual Profile of Men in Power* (James, Bess, and Saltus, 1978), the authors document extensive and extreme sadomasochistic behavior with prostitutes among contemporary American politicians in the Washington, D.C. area. The psychiatric profile on the representative individual is of a man whose messianic, addictive drive for power is based on unresolved oedipal rivalries:

> . . .in the case of those politicians who need to indulge in painful practices with call girls, does the acting out of these sadomasochistic fantasies make them more or less likely to behave in ways which may threaten the public welfare? That is, is it a principle of catharsis which is operating here, or does this behavior lead to an accumulation of pressure which eventually may cause them to lose control in situations where a disciplined rationality is essential to our very survival? On the other hand, if we were to remove such people from the political arena, would we necessarily be better off? Would we be eliminating those men who merely have a stronger political drive, correlated with a more intense sex drive, or would we perhaps be filtering out the men who make the most effective leaders?

These questions may be among the most important that mankind will ever ask. If answers are not soon forthcoming, they may also be among the last.

The psychiatric literature on sadomasochism is extensive. It is also relentlessly theoretical. These interrelated, often interconflicting theories have two essential features in common. All are unproven and nearly all describe and define S&M in a context of psychopathology. An exception is Theodore Reik's formidable intellectual treatise, *Masochism in Sex and Society* (1941). In giving such philosophical scope to the vagueness of boundary in sadomasochism, Reik, perhaps unwittingly, avoids the characterization of his subjects or their activities as abnormal. With a perspective that can appreciate Christianity — in its equating of love with submission, and its divinity of suffering and death — as a supreme expression of moral sadomasochism, Reik cautiously eschews the subtle psychoanalytic tendency towards moralizing judgment. His perception that Christ's victory-through-defeat psychology was quintessentially masochistic and that "the late Jewish prophets and the Christian faith bring the glorification of masochism," reveals his sense for the labyrinthine, perhaps infinite complexity of his subject.

By contrast, much of the psychiatric literature implicitly judges sadomasochism as it did homosexuality, on the basis of those individuals whose happiness and functioning are perceived by themselves, or defined by their environment, as being disturbed or impaired (i.e., on the basis of those individuals who are seen by the psychiatrist). In "Masochism " (*Medical Aspects of Human Sexuality,* 11/1972), Henriette Klein generalizes from her own clinical experience:

> Both the masochist and the sadist overeroticize and overemphasize sex in that sex looms out of proportion to all else in life. Both experience great anxiety with the sexual act and can never really feel free to enjoy it. They come to the act with anxiety and depart from it with added guilt.

The short step from her description of a few individuals with problems of psychological adaptation, to implicit generalization about all those whose sexual behavior includes sadomasochistic practices, is as easy as it is deceptive. Beyond the issue of extrapolation, Dr. Klein's comments obfuscate the essential features of masochism. That sadomasochists experience anxiety and guilt in their sexual communications is obvious. That "they can never really feel free to enjoy it" is superficial—far from Reik's elegant hypothesis that "in the place of pleasure accompanied by anxiety, there steps anxiety-producing pleasure, resulting in an osmosis of pleasure and anxiety." Throughout his work, Reik is at pains to stress the foundation, substance, and instinctual aim of (sado)masochism—pleasure. "Pleasure is the aim, never to be abolished, and the masochistic staging is but a circuitous way to reach this aim. The urge for pleasure is so powerful that anxiety and the idea of punishment themselves are drawn into its sphere."

Many of Reik's ideas are, of course, derived from Freud. In fact, most psychiatric expostulations on sadomasochism are minor vicissitudes of the master's instinctive theorizing on the subject. Despite his inclusion of sadomasochism among "the sexual aberrations," Freud continually notes its variable presentation in the everyday behavior of normal individuals.

> The roots of active algolagnia, sadism, can be readily demonstrable in the normal individual. The sexuality of most men shows an admixture of aggression, of a desire to subdue, the biological significance of which lies in the necessity for overcoming the resistance of the sexual

object by actions other than courting. Sadism and masochism occupy a special place in the perversions, for the contrast of activity and passivity lying at their bases belongs to the common traits of the sexual life. That cruelty and the sexual instinct are most intimately connected is beyond doubt taught by the history of civilization. The most striking peculiarity of this perversion lies in the fact that its active and passive forms are regularly encountered together in the same person (*Three Contributions to the Theory of Sex,* 1905).

The most interesting feature of Freud's thinking about sadomasochism is its uncertainty. His conclusion that it should be considered a perversion only when the condition of sexual satisfaction is entirely dependent on the humiliation and maltreatment of the sexual object, or obversely, when that satisfaction is exclusively conditional upon either physical or mental suffering, leaves a vast realm of behaviors uncharted.

Elsewhere in *Three Contributions to the Theory of Sex,* Freud describes masochism as "a perversion that seems further removed from the normal sexual goal than its opposite. It may even be doubted whether it ever is primary and whether it does not more often originate through transformation from sadism." Yet two decades later, Freud was no longer satisfied with this assumption. In some of the most controversial thinking of the twentieth century, he now proposed the existence of two primary instincts: the sexual urge, also called Eros, and the death instinct, linked with aggression ("Beyond the Pleasure Principle," 1920). The constructive tendencies of the former drive, he claimed, are opposed to the destructive tendencies of the latter. The two antagonistic fundamental urges that struggle against each other in all creation are seen to continue this battle in the life of all individuals. With this revision of his theory of instincts, Freud now believed in the existence of a primary masochism, a universal, normal tendency in all human beings towards self-destruction.

Ultimately, Freud delineated three principal manifestations of masochism. *Moral* masochism was seen to be the psychosocial complement to sexual or *feminine* masochism. The third type, *erotogenic,* was thought to be a kind of biological-constitutional foundation upon which moral and feminine masochism are constructed. (A full accounting of Freud's clearly unresolved thinking about aggression and sadomasochism is beyond the scope of this discussion. This literature is interpreted with care and perspective by Erich Fromm in *The Anatomy of Human Destructiveness* (1975) and by Shirley Panken in *The Joy of Suffering* (1973).)

Freud wrote much about the intimate relationship between masochism and femininity. Since an essential feature of masochism is surrender — submission to the sexual object — what would often be called masochism in the male is here considered to be normal sexual behavior in the female. With little semantic choreography, one might then argue that if the woman is masochistic by nature, she is not masochistic. That is, it would not be a pathological reaction so much as a natural phenomenon, a kind of secondary sex characteristic.

This is a troubling feature of the psychiatric literature. While granting that the normal female does not ordinarily see, even if she will gladly endure, pain and humiliation, masochism in the female would be designated as such only in the most extreme instances of self-destructive behavior. From this perspective, it is understandable that Freud and his adherents saw masochism as a perversion that is exceedingly rare among women. It is also understandable and most intriguing that these same thinkers saw masochism as the prevailing perversion among men.

Many feminists and gay rights activists have expressed concern that Freud's interpretation of masochism supports patriarchal mythology and prejudice; that Freud basically described feminine sexuality with negative connotations, and feminine or submissive sexuality in males as pathology.

Otto Rank, a pupil, colleague, and early follower of Freud, was later one of his chief dissenters. In *Beyond Psychology* (1941), he perceived masochism to be the culturally perpetrated result of patriarchal attitudes.

> Wide and deepened experience in the field of psychotherapy has con-
> vinced me that the ultimate "cause" of most feminine neurosis is
> modern man, with his lack of masculine qualities and his inability to
> want his woman lovingly, instead of willfully. . . . *This type, termed in
> modern psychology, "masochistic," does not represent an exaggeration
> of her natural passivity but rather the frustrated expression of her need
> to surrender, applied in a masculine fashion to herself.* (emphasis mine)

In *Psychoanalysis and Feminism* (1977), Juliet Mitchell defends Freud as having accurately described feminine psychology and sexuality in a patriarchal cultural context, really the only context in which femininity, however distorted, has ever been observed. "Entering today into what would seem to be only a revamped patriarchal society, the little girl has to acquire, and quickly too, her cultural destiny, which is made to appear misleadingly coincident with a biological one." What becomes increasingly clear from the literature is that sadomasochism, like femininity, is to a large extent culturally defined.

In the intervening years since Freud, the psychiatric interpretations of sadism and masochism, like the patriarchy of evolving Western civilization, have changed little. The American Psychiatric Association's *1980 Diagnostic Manual of Mental Disorders* (DSM-III) . . . described "sexual masochism" as far more common among males. Likewise, "sexual sadism occurs far more frequently in males than in females. The more severe forms of the condition are virtually never seen in females." Although the limited sex research data are congruent with the psychiatric view of male predominance in sadomasochism, the data are by no means conclusive. As noted in the Spengler study, female participation would be expected to be, and doubtless is, far more socioculturally inhibited. Even so, in both New York and San Francisco, female involvement is growing, and San Francisco actually has three clubs whose members are exclusively female.

Could the tendency to anticipate and experience sexual pleasure in association with the suffering or inflicting of physical pain be a component of healthy sexuality? In their chapter on "painful stimulation techniques" (*Patterns of Sexual Behavior,* 1951), anthropologists Ford and Beach think so.

> Societies in which intercourse is regularly associated with biting, scratching or hair pulling prove inevitably to be the ones in which children and adolescents are allowed a great deal of sexual freedom. Furthermore, if the cultural stereotype of satisfactory intercourse includes a considerable amount of moderately painful interaction, it also represents the woman as an active, vigorous participant in all things sexual.

The sexual connection between pleasure and pain may well be more biological than psychological or cultural. During the last decade, a mysterious group of internally manufactured, opiate-like substances called "endorphins" has been identified and isolated. Like their synthetically created analogues, the narcotics (heroin, morphine, and their derivatives), the endorphins effect an indifference to physical and mental suffering, and a profound sense of well-being. These substances are released in the brain and throughout the central nervous system in response to various stresses and noxious or painful stimuli. They are believed to be the mechanism responsible for pain relief in acupuncture and may be what stimulates the ecstasies so often described by religious flagellants and martyrs.

These substances are perhaps also released during hypnosis. New York psychiatrist Paul Sacerdote has speculated that endorphins may be responsible for the analgesia in minor surgical procedures wherein hypnosis is the sole anesthetic agent. Although recent experiments have failed to substantiate this hypothesis, a possible relationship between endorphins and hypnotic phenomena has not been ruled out.

Various degrees of hypnosis are believed to be involved in the calming, euphoriant effects of religious ritual and ceremony. Hypnosis of the self (auto-hypnosis) is the state of tranquility that one seeks in meditation or prayer. Hypnosis between leader and subject is probably what transpires during catholic confession, faith-healing, the state of being in love, effective psychotherapy, and mob behavior. That a kind of pain relief might be the basis for patriotism and its companions, religious zealotry and xenophobia, is intriguing.

Like heroin and morphine, the endorphins have recently been discovered to be addictive. Perhaps the incorporation of pain into sexual activity is actually a mechanism for releasing or augmenting the release of these sub-stances in the brain. If this is true, the fact that many have observed sado-masochistic behavior to be progressive (the sadomasochist may have a tendency to become involved in progressively "heavier" scenes) would be consistent with this addictive potential of the endorphins. It would also be consistent with Reik's observation that the masochist is a pleasure-seeker whose plea-sure appears to be of incomparable character, intensity, and duration. Pain, in other words, is possibly a mechanism of addiction to pleasure.

To say that psychiatry is unanimous in designating all sadomasochistic behavior as intrinsically pathologic would be erroneous. The DSM-III that characterizes sadism and masochism as almost exclusively male perversions also qualifies that tendencies in both directions can be components of normal sexuality. In fairness, it must be emphasized that when psychiatry defines such a behavior as disordered, it is not always proposing a blanket value judgment of the behavior so much as describing the dystonicity that results for the affected individual in the context of paternal and sociocultural value systems. Suicide is an example of this. In Western cultures, suicidal ten-dencies are almost universally regarded as pathologic. In the East, however, suicidal ideation may be considered as appropriate responses to such circumstances as defeat or infidelity.

Homosexuality is an example of a deviation that in our culture is often ego-dystonic. That is, while no longer considered by official psychiatry to be pathological in and of itself, homosexuality may be rendered ego-dystonic by sociocultural proscriptions. The affected individual, having internalized these mores, may as a result be incapable of a positive acceptance of what may well turn out to be his biologic (genetic) self. In 1973, the American Psychiatric Association (APA), bowing to the impressive findings of sex researchers in consonance with psychiatry's own history of persistent failure in therapeutic efforts to change established homosexual orientations, removed homosexuality from its list of mental disorders. In the DSM-III description of "ego-dystonic homosexuality," there is the remarkable capitulation that much of this dystonicity is sociogenic.

Nevertheless, many psychiatrists still dispute the 1973 APA ruling. Most are orthodox psychoanalysts who still consider homosexuality to be, *univer-sally,* a retardation of personality maturation, arrested in various stages of psychosexual development. Because homosexuality is thought by such psychiatrists to be intrinsically infantile ("narcissistic"), it is also believed to sustain an intimate relationship to sadomasochism (in the paradigms of psychoanalysis, an expression of infantile sexual drives and conflicts); in much the same way that (sado)masochism has been thought, by analogous analytic reasoning, to sustain an intimate relationship to femininity.

These psychiatrists, Dr. Socarides outstanding among them, lend "moral" support to the erotophobic fears and accusations of sexual igno-rance. To what should be their professional shame and censure, they lend little else. Socarides, with the others, has persistently failed to reproduce the "cures" he claims to be both possible and necessary for this "serious disorder." Following a long tradition of psychoanalysts from Freud to Anna Freud, from Bergler to Bieber to Hatterer, Socarides has viewed the cross-gender identifications and erotosexual bonding of homosexuality as expressions of infantile sadomasochistic conflicts. *Homosexuality* (1978), a political resurrection of his earlier work, *The Overt Homosexual* (1968), is an eerie measure of the distance psychoanalytic psychiatry has "advanced" in the sexual revolution. Here, therapeutic results are only twice accounted for, as follows: 1) "A definitive breakdown and analysis of the therapeutic results is currently being written" (p. 406); 2) "A Ten-Year Follow-Up Interview with a Successfully Treated Patient." This is a transcription of a taped interview with one of the "cures" (p. 497).

Generally speaking, psychiatry is Janus-faced about sadomasochism. On the one hand, moral and sexual sadomasochistic patterns are regularly and confidently analyzed through oedipal microscopes. On the other, there are sometimes vague, fleeting concessions to the existence of a primary constitutional masochism. How important is this "primary masochism"? And if it is ubiquitous, as Freud oscillatingly believed, how is it manifested in the "mature" personality?

This ambivalence is a prominent feature of *A Prince of Our Disorder* (1976), Harvard psychiatrist John Mack's psychobiography of T. E. Lawrence (of Arabia). While emphasizing Lawrence's powerful identification with his guilt-ridden mother and the childhood experience of being severely and repeatedly beaten by her, he also adds that Lawrence may have been suffering from "a biologically rooted masochistic predisposition."

It is pertinent to recall that T. E. Lawrence, one of British history's greatest military leaders, was throughout his years of achievement an unconscious, asexual sadomasochist. In their work with sexually dysfunctional couples, Masters and Johnson have stressed the titanic influence of religions and their associated cultural and political moralities in the genesis of crippled sexuality. "There is no question about it. Unequivocally, absolutely, religious orthodoxy (whether Jewish, Catholic or Protestant) is responsible for a significant degree of sexual dysfunction." As with Lawrence, whether religious or culturally inspired sexual abstinence diminishes, facilitates, or perverts beneficial achievement is unknown. It is a matter for speculation. It is thus most urgently a matter for investigative inquiry.

In *Beyond Sexual Freedom,* Dr. Charles Socarides discusses the implications of the sexual revolution:

> Man's crucial failure is that he has been unable to manage the "beast" within himself. He has been unable to collect and integrate inner knowledge in order to employ it in the capacity of love, for understanding the gratification of his instinctual needs in a way beneficial to

himself and to society. When he regresses to the level of emotional thought, brute emotion, or even lower and further back in his primitive past to sheer hedonic response (of either elemental pain or pleasure), technology becomes a dangerous toy in the hands of the beast of pride.

But if man is never allowed to regress to the level of emotional thought or brute emotion or sheer hedonic response in the form of controlled, consensual fantasy, what happens to these impulses? Where do they go? How do they become gratified? Socarides, at the level of Bryant and Briggs, would argue that "the beast" within man must somehow be employed "in the capacity for love."

Gore Vidal recently reflected during a discussion of "born-again" Christianity, "When I hear the word *love,* I reach for my revolver." Does he suspect the "beast"? Has he seen other faces of Janus' love? The love of God, perhaps, as expressed in the Crusades, the inquisitions, the witch burnings of Europe and of Salem, or the suicides of Guyana? Or the love of country and countryman as manifested by such patriots as Hitler, Stalin, and Idi Amin? Or the love of man and his family as annunciated by the likes of John Briggs, Anita Bryant, and Reverend Jim Jones . . . and Dr. Charles Socarides?

Perhaps Mr. Vidal suspects that the gratification of bestial impulses in the vestments of *love* has resulted in nothing less than the atrocity-ridden history and possible future of "civilization."

*Recommended reading list has been deleted from the original article. Lawrence Mass's reference to Susanne P. Schad-Somers's book (p. 48 above) pertains to *Sadomasochism,* Human Sciences Press, 1982.—*Eds.*

Andreas Spengler

Manifest Sadomasochism of Males
Results of an Empirical Study

INTRODUCTION

Manifest sadomasochism among men has previously been described in the scientific literature only as a perversion or as an individual pathological phenomenon, not as a problem with social implications. One finds studies which describe only clinical aspects. The manner in which sadomasochists deal with their sexual needs and realize their desires, as well as the social and psychic consequences of their orientation, remains unknown.

In his article "Fetishism and Sadomasochism," Gebhard (1969) emphasized how widespread this deviation is: "these quantitative aspects fully justify fetishism and sadomasochism receiving more attention" and "in our present state of knowledge [we] cannot offer any reasoned theories buttressed by factual data."

An exploratory and primarily descriptive study concerning the social situation and the sexual behavior of heterosexual, bisexual, and homosexual men with a manifestly sadomasochistic orientation was designed. In the course of the study, our special interest was devoted to the subcultural forms in which they are organized, possibilities for realizing the deviant behavior, and finally the consequences that arise in the course of working out the social conflicts which derive from the deviance.

We define manifest sadomasochistic deviance as a specialization of a type of sexual behavior where the interaction between the partners is concentrated on inflicting and receiving physical and psychic pain, or on ritualized submission and dominance. We define subcultures as social systems in

Reprinted from *Archives of Sexual Behavior*, Vol. 6, No. 6, 1977: 441–456. Copyright © 1977 by Plenum Publishing Corporation. Reprinted by permission of the publisher and the author.

which special norms of behavior are valid that deviate from the norms of the superimposed social system, used as a point of reference, and that make possible the deviant behavior. Where the sadomasochistic practice is affirmed and such partnerships are made possible, a social arena is created in which the usual stigmatization of sadomasochistic behavior is suspended and is partially replaced by a positive counternorm. The independence of subcultural systems is evidenced by forms of communication peculiar to them (for example, specific linguistic systems and nonverbal rules of communication) and by special social institutions (Arnold, 1970).

METHOD

Extreme difficulties exist in questioning sadomasochists. Heterosexual sadomasochists live undercover; their groups are cut off from the outside world. The existence of subcultural groups among them has been doubted (Simon and Gagnon, 1970; Hunt, 1970). Only homosexual sadomasochists appeared to be approachable for investigation (Dannecker and Reiche, 1974). Anonymity is one of the special norms of sadomasochistic subcultures.

These conditions were taken into account by carrying out the study using a questionnaire to be filled out anonymously. Subjects were reached in two ways:

1. We sent questionnaires in response to contact advertisements used by sadomasochists to seek partners.
2. We had questionnaires distributed to members by cooperating sadomasochistic clubs.

(If one desires to go beyond individual case studies and studies of sadomasochistic prostitution, it is almost impossible to question sadomasochistically oriented women in the subculture; there are hardly any nonprostitute ads and very few women in the clubs. As a result, we investigated men only.) We distributed 877 questionnaires (44% by contact ads, 56% by clubs). Responses were received from 245 men. The response rate was 27% for the ads, 29% for the club members, and 28% for the total.

In the definitive sample, heterosexual and homosexual sadomasochists were to be represented approximately equally. It turned out that a bisexual choice of partners was usual. We therefore divided the sample into three approximately equal groups: persons with an exclusively heterosexual choice of partners (30%), those with a bisexual choice (31%), and those with an exclusively homosexual one (38%) (see Table I). There are two effects of the selection which could have influenced the results:

1. With respect to the population of all sadomasochists, obtaining the sample by means of subcultural clubs or contact ads represents a limitation: only persons who share their deviance with others somewhere, be it only in an anonymous ad, are accounted for.

2. The response rate of 27% constitutes a selection in which those might well be overrepresented who are open and self-confident about their deviance (as indicated by their readiness to participate). A comparison of the contents of the contact ads of the persons who returned the questionnaire with those of the persons who withheld a response yielded good agreement in the basic variables of the heterosexual-bisexual-homosexual orientation and of the active-passive orientation of sadomasochistic roles.

Table I.   Sexual Orientation of Male Sadomasochists
(self-rating, n = 244)

Orientation	Percent
Exclusively heterosexual	30
Bisexual, more heterosexual	11
Bisexual	4
Bisexual, more homosexual	16
Exclusively homosexual	38

Table II.   Demographic Data for Male Sadomasochists

a. Age (n = 240)	Percent
25 years or younger	10
26–30 years	14
31–40 years	34
41–50 years	20
51 years or older	21

b. Education (n = 244)	Percent
9 years of school (Hauptschulabschluss)	37
10 years of school (Mittlere Reife)	22
13 years of school (Abitur)	15
University (postgraduate)	25

c. Monthly net earnings (Deutsche Marks)[a]	Percent
No answer	9
1000 DM or less	16
Up to 1500 DM	21
Up to 2000 DM	24
2000 DM or more	30

[a]In the Federal Republic, 34% of the employed men had a net income of more than 1400 Deutsche Marks per month in 1974.

Our sample consequently included men who sought sadomasochistic partnerships via ads or clubs, participated in subcultural media of communication, and were prepared to take part in an anonymous written questionnaire investigation concerning their sexual behavior. In the sample, the upper age groups were overrepresented. There were no persons younger than 20 years of age. The individuals often had a high social status, lived in good circumstances, and were well educated (Table II). The heterosexual, bisexual, and homosexual subgroups do not differ significantly with respect to these demographic characteristics. The fact that persons with a higher social status were so heavily represented might be attributable to the effects of the selection in obtaining the sample. Subcultural realization of the deviance could be easier for persons having more disposable time and money; the better-educated could be more motivated to participate in the investigation.

RESULTS

Invisibility

The social situation of sadomasochists is characterized by the necessity of keeping the deviant behavior a secret from the outside world (Table III). Mother, father, sister, and brother often know nothing about it. An especially difficult situation occurs in marriage: the deviant desires are frequently incompatible with the interests of the wife, and many of the wives are not informed about the deviance. The divorce rate in our sample was above average, 16% among heterosexuals, 12% among bisexuals, and 5% among homosexuals.

Table III. Invisibility of the Sadomasochistic Behavior

	Knows of suspects it (%)	Does not know (%)	No answer (%)
Mother (n = 176)	19	66	15
Father (n = 150)	9	69	23
Brother, sister (n = 182)	15	65	19
Wife (n = 109)	35	41	24

	Many (%)	Some (%)	None (%)	No answer (%)
Friends (n = 245)	7	47	41	4
Colleagues (n = 245)	2	9	70	18

Seeking a Partner

Most of the sadomasochists studied used contact advertisements: only 7% had never placed an ad, and only 14% were advertising for the first time on the occasion of the investigation. The number of responses to the last ad (Table IVa) is a good indicator of the chance of finding a partner in this manner. Heterosexual sadomasochists had less opportunity to make contacts via ads than did homosexuals. Among the latter, only 4% received no response, but the rate was 25% among heterosexuals. The contact ads were the most frequently employed method to make contact (Table IVb); the other means of making contact are relevant only for subgroups and vary with sexual orientation. For example, information from friends, pubs, bars, and parties were named more frequently by homosexuals, while heterosexuals more often cited prostitution as their source. Homosexuals and bisexuals as well had significantly better possibilities for making contact than heterosexuals (Table IVc): in 20% of the cases the latter had "become acquainted with no partner at all" with whom they could have sadomasochistic sex. This was the case with only 6% of the bisexuals and 4% of the homosexuals.

Participation in the Subculture

Sadomasochists are integrated into their subcultural groups to various degrees, and their participation in the subculture likewise varies. Subcultural integration can be measured by active participation in subcultural activities such as sadomasochistic parties (Table Va). Approximately one-third mentioned this. An "acquaintance with like-minded persons" who also had "S/M interests" existed in 59% of the cases (Table Vb). Relatively fewer heterosexual sadomasochists participated in these direct subcultural contacts. All the more important are the indirect forms of participation in subcultural activities. Sadomasochistic correspondence is a widespread form of communication, which often includes sexual excitement. Only one-fifth of the persons studied had not made use of this (Table Vc). The purchase of sadomasochistic literature or pornographic magazines can also serve this function, especially when contact ads are listed by these media. Most sadomasochists purchase these media regularly or frequently (Table Vd).

Possibilities for Realizing the Deviance

The frequency of sadomasochistic experiences with partners in the last 12 months was low in the sample: only one in five had such an experience weekly, 15% had none at all. At about 5 per year, the median frequency is

Table IV. Seeking a Sadomasochistic Partner

a. Number of responses to the last advertisement placed (%)

	Total (n=225)	Heterosexual (n=73)	Bisexual (n=71)	Homosexual (n=81)	p
No answer	14	25	14	4	
1–5 answers	44	42	34	56	
6–10 answers	20	18	24	18	0.01
More answers	22	15	28	22	

b. Ways in which a sadomasochistic sex partner was found (%)

	Total (n=244)	Heterosexual (n=74)	Bisexual (n=77)	Homosexual (n=93)	p
Contact ads	64	51	80	60	0.001
Friends	36	24	31	49	0.002
Pubs	25	15	25	33	0.05
Special bars	23	15	19	33	0.02
Parks	21	4	27	31	0.001
Clubs	20	12	23	25	n.s.
Prostitution	13	23	9	7	0.01
Parties	8	3	10	12	n.s.

c. "No partner at all" for sadomasochistic sex (%)

	Total (n=244)	Heterosexual (n=74)	Bisexual (n=77)	Homosexual (n=93)	p
	10	20	6	4	0.001

relatively low. In the total sample the number of partners (4.5 per year) is scarcely lower and from this we can conclude that the sexual forms of behavior of sadomasochism are characterized by low frequency and a relatively great number of partners. Table VI shows further that homosexuals and bisexuals have better possibilities of realization than heterosexuals. The latter had on the average 3.3 contacts with 2.8 partners in the last 12 months; homosexual sadomasochists by contrast had 5.7 contacts with 7.0 partners; the bisexual group had frequencies and partner numbers similar to those of the homosexuals. Significant differences occur among the groups in the case of frequency of contacts as well as in partner numbers.

The question concerning length of last relationship with a sadomasochistic partner yielded widely varying answers. Half who had had such a relationship (n=182) had it for over a year; however, 14% had a relationship for less than a week. This was observed to be independent of sexual

Table V.   Participation in the Sadomasochistic Subculture

a. Subcultural integration: "How often do you meet with like-minded persons for S/M parties (last 12 months)" (%)

	Total (n = 244)	Heterosexual (n = 74)	Bisexual (n = 77)	Homosexual (n = 93)	p
Never	67	85	57	60	
1–5 times	20	12	23	25	0.001
More often	13	3	19	14	

b. Acquaintance with like-minded persons: "Do you have acquaintances with S/M interests?" (%)

	Total (n = 224)	Heterosexual (n = 74)	Bisexual (n = 77)	Homosexual (n = 93)	p
Yes	59	34	57	81	
No	41	66	43	19	0.001

c. Sadomasochistic correspondence (last 12 months) (%)

	Total (n = 245)	
Never	21	
Sometimes	54	(no significant difference among
Often	25	subgroups)

d. Purchase of sadomasochistic magazines (last 12 months) (%)

	Total (n = 230)	
Never	0	
1 time	9	
2–5 times	21	
6–25 times	54	(no significant difference among
More often	15	subgroups)

orientation. Several questions were directed at the form of partnership (firm relationship, loose relationship, prostitution) in which sadomasochistic experiences are possible. The following observations resulted (Table VIc): loose partnerships predominated over firm relationships, only slightly in partnerships with women but considerably in partnerships with men. By contrast, prostitution played a subordinate role, except for possible sadomasochistic experiences with a woman. The respective partnerships with active and passive sadomasochistic activities were named with practically the same frequency (with the exception of heterosexual prostitution), because for the most part active and passive role divisions occur together in a partnership.

Table VI.   Possibilities for Realizing the Sadomasochistic Deviance

a. Frequency of sadomasochistic sex with partners (last 12 months) (%)

	Total (n = 238)	Heterosexual (n = 74)	Bisexual (n = 76)	Homosexual (n = 88)	p
Never	15	26	12	8	
1–3 times	20	26	20	16	
4–6 times	28	24	24	34	0.01
7–24 times	19	15	25	17	
More often	18	9	20	25	

b. Number of sadomasochistic sex partners (last 12 months) (%)

	Total (n = 244)	Heterosexual (n = 74)	Bisexual (n = 77)	Homosexual (n = 93)	p
0	5	13	0	3	
1	11	14	13	6	
2–3	25	36	18	20	0.001
4–5	21	22	26	16	
6–10	15	13	17	16	
More	23	1	26	38	

c. Sadomasochistic activities in different partnerships[a] (%)

	Steady partner	Loose partner	Prostitute
Heterosexual			
Active sadistic activities (n = 66 partnerships)[a]	38	47	15
Passive masochistic activities (n = 63 partnerships)[a]	30	35	35
Homosexual			
Active sadistic activities (n = 102 partnerships)[a]	27	65	7
Passive masochistic activities (n = 105 partnerships)[a]	25	65	10

[a]Since each partner engages in active and passive activities side by side in many partnerships, the data given here overlap.

In summary we conclude that the bisexual group has possibilities for realizing its sadomasochistic desires that are nearly as good as those of the homosexual group. The chances of the heterosexuals are significantly less. This might be interpreted to mean that the inclusion of men as partners for

Table VII.   Self-acceptance of Sadomasochists

---

a. Judgment of one's own sexual orientation
    (n = 245) (%)

"It's different from the ordinary, but all right"	78
"Many more people ought to be like this"	49
"That is absolutely normal"	41
"That is burdening"	20
"That is morbid"	3
"It's immoral"	1

b. Emotional reactions after sadomasochistic sex
    (n = 220) (%)

"I want to do it again"	85
"It was fun"	84
"It was sexually satisfying"	79
"I feel happy"	53
"I have a bad conscience"	6
"I've got to quit this"	6
"I am depressed"	4
"I regret it"	4

c. General acceptance of the sadomasochistic
    deviation: "If you could decide freely which
    sexual disposition you wanted to have, what
    would you be?" (%)

Rejection of sadomasochistic orientation	20
Acceptation of the deviant orientation	70
Don't know	9

d. Visiting a doctor, psychiatrist, or psychologist
    because of the sadomasochistic deviation (%)

Never	90
At least once	10

e. Attempt to commit suicide (%)

Never	91
At least once	9

---

sadomasochistic practice can often occur as a substitute solution. Sex, but not sadomasochistic practice, is often possible with one's wife or steady partner. Loose sadomasochistic contacts with male partners often exist parallel to the firm partnership. (Similarly, among many homosexuals there are loose sadomasochistic relationships side by side with a firm nonsadomasochistic one.)

Self-acceptance

According to our hypothesis, direct or indirect integration into the deviant subculture makes possible the mitigation of conflicts arising from the deviant sexual orientation and poor acceptance of these desires. Interpretations of interaction theory concerning sexual subcultures point in this direction (Plummer, 1975). We thus expect that many persons in our sample (characterized by a relatively active subcultural integration) would have a positive relation to their deviance. We tried to measure self-acceptance in several questions. Regarding one's own self-judgment and emotional reactions after sadomasochistic experiences, positive ratings (for example, "it's perfectly normal" or "it was fun") predominated over negative ones (for example, "it's sick" or "I've got to get out of this"). Moreover, most would want to be sadomasochists even if they could "decide freely about it" (Table VIIc). Only 10% had seen a doctor or psychiatrist because of their sadomasochistic deviance (Table VIId), and 9% had tried to commit suicide (Table VIIe) (with few exceptions these two groups are not identical). The rate of attempted suicides is less than that of homosexual men in West Germany (Dannecker and Reiche, 1974). Thus only a minority in our sample appeared not to have found a way to positive self-acceptance; only about one-fifth responded with a gross negative reaction. We found a number of significant correlations which indicate that subcultural integration (defined by the frequency of participation in sadomasochistic parties) and the possibility of realizing the deviance in a partnership context are associated with self-acceptance. Positive self-judgments and positive emotional reactions after deviant experiences (for example "I'm happy" or "many more people ought to be like this") was affirmed significantly more frequently by active participants in the subculture. This confirms our hypothesis that having social roots in the subculture decisively influences the possibility of a positive self-acceptance.

Sadomasochistic Role Orientation

Only a minority of our sample were oriented in an exclusively active (sadistic) or passive (masochistic) direction (Table VIII). Most sadomasochists, heterosexuals as well as homosexuals, alternate between these roles. In this manner they can adapt themselves more flexibly to different partners. At the same time varying preferences for one or the other of the two roles can be realized. Consequently, we speak of preferences for certain roles in sadomasochistic interaction which we designate as active, versatile, and passive sadomasochistic role orientation. Our statistical analysis reveals only few significant differences among persons with a more active role orientation, a versatile one, or a more passive one. The social and sexual

Table VIII.   Sadomasochistic Role Orientation (%)[a,b]

Orientation	Total (n = 243)	Heterosexual (n = 73)	Bisexual (n = 76)	Homosexual (n = 93)
Exclusively active	13	16	12	12
Versatile, mainly active	19	19	20	18
Versatile	29	23	28	37
Versatile, mainly passive	22	16	30	20
Exclusively passive	16	25	10	13

[a]p = n.s.
[b]Answer to the question: "Do you prefer the active role (lord, master, teacher) or the passive role (servant, slave, pupil) in S/M sex?"

behavior is not dependent on this role preference. The fact of assuming an active or passive role with a partner is, therefore, of no decisive consequence for the realization of this deviation.

Degree of Preference for Sadomasochistic Practices

In the article referred to previously, Gebhard (1969) emphasized that fetishism is a "graduated phenomenon." This can also be applied to sadomasochism. We define the degree of preference by the frequency with which sadomasochistic practices are desired in sexual experience. In this sense, an exclusive preference was reported by 16% of the subjects. The group of those who only occasionally desired to include sadomasochistic elements in their experiences was likewise 16%. Medium preferences and strong but not exclusive preferences each amounted to 32% (Table IXa). An exclusive fixation on deviant practices is thus relatively rare. This may also be observed in the fact that only 15% could experience an orgasm exclusively with sadomasochistic activities. By contrast, 45% experienced orgasm without any sadomasochistic activity (Table IXb). Heterosexuals, bisexuals, and homosexuals do not vary in this respect. There was a somewhat stronger fixation on these practices by the passively oriented persons (Table IXa).

Sadomasochistic Practices

Table X summarizes the most widespread sadomasochistic practices and elements of fetishistic or fetish-like style. In contrast to the "classical" style elements of beating and bondage, the more extreme and actually dangerous practices occurred with minimal frequency. A distinction between various types of behavior such as "hardcore S/M" and "flagellism" (or the divisions

Table IX.   Degree of Sadomasochistic Preference

a. Preferred relative frequency of sadomasochistic sex with respect to the sadomasochistic role (%)

	Total (n = 239)	Active (n = 77)	Versatile (n = 69)	Passive (n = 92)	p
"I would like sex. . .					
exclusively with S/M"	16	13	3	29	
predominantly with S/M"	32	30	36	33	
equally often with and without S/M"	32	35	42	23	0.001
predominantly without S/M"	16	22	19	15	
only without S/M"	2[a]	—	—	—	

b. Conditions of orgasm: "Under what conditions do you come to sexual climax with a partner?" (n = 245) (%)

without sadomasochistic activity	45
with sadomasochistic activity	79
with sadomasochistic fantasies	44
exclusively with sadomasochistic activity	15

[a]These persons were primarily oriented fetishistically.

Table X.   Sadomasochistic Practices and Fetishistic Preference (n = 233)

Practice	Percent
Cane	60
Whip	66
Bonds	60
Anal manipulations	26
"Torture" apparatus	27
Nipple torture	9
Needles	6
Clothespins/clamps	7
Glowing objects	7
Knives/razor blades	4

Fetishistic preference	Percent
Leather	50
Boots	50
Jeans	19
Uniforms	16
"Strafhose"	11
Rubber	12
Women's clothing	14
Urolagnia	10
Coprophilia	5
"Dirty sex"	3

between "bondage" and "spanking," etc., common in the United States) appears to be inconsequential with respect to the social and sexual situation.

As described elsewhere, fetishistic preferences to the point of definite fixations on certain fetishes (in our sample among about one-third) are widespread. (This group revealed no practical difference from the remaining sadomasochists.) We also found hardly any relevant differences among the practices of homosexual, bisexual, or heterosexual sadomasochists.

Masturbation

The relationship of masturbation frequencies and sexual orientation was studied. Such a comparison must first of all be based on the observation that heterosexual and homosexual men have highly varying masturbation frequencies. The comparison in our sample showed no significant difference among heterosexual, bisexual, and homosexual sadomasochists (Table XI). A comparison with the data of Dannecker and Reiche (1974) reveals that the frequencies we observed are approximately as high as those of the "common homosexuals" in West Germany. Similar to the findings of Dannecker and Reiche, the highest masturbation frequencies in our sample occurred among persons who had deviant experiences with partners most frequently. It would therefore be shortsighted to view the high masturbation frequencies as substitute satisfaction. It is rather a question of a behavior which exists independently alongside the partnership forms of sadomasochistic practice. This becomes clear in the frequency of autoerotic sadomasochistic activities: 28% reported self-bondage, self-beating, torture of nipples with clamps, and the like during masturbation.

Coming Out

We define the first awareness of sadomasochistic desires as "sadomasochistic coming out." Table XIIa shows that this experience occurred relatively

Table XI.   Frequency of Masturbation (last 12 months) (%)[a]

Frequency	Total (n = 244)	Heterosexual (n = 74)	Bisexual (n = 77)	Homosexual (n = 93)
Never	4	8	4	1
Less than once per month	12	15	13	9
About once per month	14	13	17	12
About once per week	18	16	16	21
More than once per week	38	36	32	45
Daily	13	11	18	12

[a]p = n.s.

Table XII.   Sadomasochistic Coming Out

a. Age of the first awareness of sadomasochistic desires: "How old were you when you realized for the first time that you had a special sexual preference or disposition for S/M?" (n = 237) (%)

	Total (n = 237)	Heterosexual (n = 70)	Bisexual (n = 77)	Homosexual (n = 90)	p
10 years or younger	7	11	5	6	
11 to 13 years	10	10	10	11	
14 to 16 years	25	21	26	26	
17 to 19 years	15	21	9	13	n.s.
20 to 24 years	20	23	18	18	
25 to 29 years	12	6	16	16	
30 years or older	11	7	16	11	

b. Emotional reactions to the coming out: ". . . How did you react to it?" (n = 245) (%)

"I was glad"	24
"I felt happy"	22
"I was proud"	13
"I wanted to do it again"	69
"I was troubled"	40
"I thought it was immoral"	23
"I was afraid about the future"	21
"I felt guilty"	11
"I was disgusted with myself"	6

late among many of the subjects: 43% experienced it only after the age of 19 years, 11% at the age of 30 or later. The portion of those who experienced their sadomasochistic coming out after the age of 25 was significantly less in the heterosexual group (13%) than in the bisexual group (32%) or the homosexual group (27%). Under the special conditions of integration into the homosexual subculture, sadomasochistic desires often appear to occur when homosexuality is already being actively practiced. In comparison with the average homosexual coming out (Dannecker and Reicher, 1974), sadomasochistic coming out occurred much later (in the homosexual group of our sample).

The first awareness of sadomasochistic desires brings a difficult conflict situation. Nevertheless, a portion of the persons we studied coped in a rather positive manner (Table XIIb). Reactions like "glad," "happy," and "proud" were affirmed much more often by those persons actively integrated into the subculture (frequent attendance of parties).

CONCLUSION

The existence of sadomasochistic subcultures (especially heterosexual ones) has heretofore been denied in sex research. Only homosexual sadomasochistic subcultural groups have been described (Gregersen, 1969; Dannecker and Reiche, 1974). As a result of the findings of our study and observations made beyond the study based on the questionnaire, this must be corrected.

Several important aspects of subcultural activity could not be measured directly through the questionnaire investigation. Our understanding of these data was expanded as a result of supplementary investigations concerning subcultural documents (for example, through an analysis of 344 advertisements of male sadomasochists, through a secondary analysis of three questionnaires of a sadomasochistic organization submitted to 270 heterosexual and homosexual club members), and on the basis of correspondence (n = 76 letters) and 15 detailed interviews with members of sadomasochistic clubs. These impressions were further expanded by the study of subcultural media (newspapers, pornography, magazines) and literature (e.g., Mechler, 1959/1960; Greene and Greene, 1974; Townsend, 1972; Schertel, 1957).

Tentative assumptions which have not yet been secured by data will be summarized. The various possibilities of finding partners who are available to heterosexual sadomasochists on the one hand and to bisexual/homosexual ones on the other, and also the varying characterization of their subcultural groups, appear to be explained by the fact that there are few women who seek this practice in the realm of the subculture. According to available data from representative studies (Kinsey et al., 1953; Hunt, 1970), there appear to be a number of women interested in sadomasochistic themes. However, the number of women prepared to enter sadomasochistic relationships in the mode of behavior that manifestly sadomasochistic men seek appears to be extremely small. This is confirmed by Nacht (1948), Deutsch (1959), and Gebhard (1969).

We consider the assumption that manifest sadomasochistic deviance among women is very rare (at least within the subculture) to be essential for an understanding of the situation of heterosexual sadomasochists. Accordingly, sadomasochistic prostitution, which in part affords the sole possibility for realization of the deviance for this group, plays a special role. With regard to our unsystematic impressions, nearly all the subcultural groups among heterosexual sadomasochists exist in cooperation with prostitutes (Bornemann, 1974). It is therefore also an important function of the heterosexually oriented subculture with its media, modes of behavior, and ideologies to maintain specifications which are supposed to make the lack of like-minded and "passionate" female partners bearable (for example, the fiction that the prostitute is indeed a genuine "sadist"). Against this background it becomes more comprehensible why the possibilities of subcultural meetings in homosexually oriented groups are far better: here a basic partner problem arising from the sex of the partner does not exist.

REFERENCES

Arnold, D. O. (1970). *Subcultures,* Glendessary Press, Berkeley, Calif.

Bornemann, E. (1974). *Sex im Volksmund I/II,* Rowolt, Reinbek/Hamburg.

Dannecker, M., and Reiche, R. (1974). *Der gewohnliche Homosexuelle,* Fischer, Frankfurt.

Deutsch, H. (1959). *Psychologie der Frau,* Huber, Bern.

Gebhard, P. H. (1969). "Fetishism and Sadomasochism." In Massermann, M. E. (Ed.), *Dynamics of Deviant Sexuality,* Grune and Stratton, New York.

Greene, G., and Greene, C. (1974). *S/M: The Last Taboo,* Grove Press, New York.

Gregersen, E. A. (1969). "The Sadomasochistic Scene." Paper read at the meeting of the American Anthropological Association.

Hunt, M. (1970). *Sexual Behavior in the 1970s,* Playboy Press, New York.

Kinsey, A. C., Pomeroy, W. B., Martin, C. E. and Gebhard, P. H. (1953). *Sexual Behavior in the Human Female,* Saunders, Philadelphia.

Mechler, U. (1959/1960). *Sadistinnen und Masochisten I/II.* Prehm, Dachau.

Nacht, S. (1948). *Le Masochisme,* Paris.

Plummer, K. (1975). *Sexual Stigma,* Routledge and Kegan Paul, London.

Schertel, E. (1957). *Flagellantismus,* Vols. 1-12, Decker, Schmiden b. Stuttgart.

Simon, W., and Gagnon, J. H. (1970). *Sexuelle Aussenseiter,* Reinbeck/Hamburg.

Townsend, L. (1972). *The Leatherman's Handbook,* The Other Traveller, New York.

G. W. Levi Kamel

The Leather Career:
On Becoming a Sadomasochist

If little is known about the origins of homosexual and heterosexual feelings in human beings, probably less is known about the emergence of sadomasochistic desires. * This ignorance is not the result of a lack of interest in this phenomenon. On the contrary, the writings of many of the greatest sexologists and personality theorists contain speculations about sadomasochism.

One of the first such works was authored by the nineteenth-century neuropsychiatrist, Richard von Krafft-Ebing, for whom sadomasochism held an intense fascination. In *Psychopathia Sexualis,* his most popular book, first published in the 1880s, he identified the psychology of women as a primary source of sadomasochistic impulses. Specifically, he suggested that sadism in males was probably "developed by the natural shyness and modesty of woman towards the aggressive manners of the male . . . particularly where the husband is hypersexual." In other words, sadistic desires develop in oversexed men who court sexually or emotionally distant women. Krafft-Ebing further wrote that, "the facts of masochism are certainly among the most interesting in the domain of psychopathology . . . (masochism) represents a pathological degeneration of the distinctive psychical peculiarities of woman." Here he says that masochism originates from a sort of frenzied female psyche. Yet, Krafft-Ebing's speculations do not explain sadomasochism without the female influence, as with gay male S&M.

*This paper is a revised version of parts of "Leathersex: Meaningful Aspects of Gay Sadomasochism," which originally appeared in *Deviant Behavior: An Interdisciplinary Journal* 1: 171-191, 1980. An edited version of the remainder of that article appears in the section on "Synthesis" in the present volume. Reprinted by permission of the author.

In his early writings, Sigmund Freud also considered sadomasochism to be a pathology. Years later, however, he refined his thinking on the topic. He came to view sadistic tendencies as an extension of the pleasure principle, an understandable, if extreme, instance of the sexual urge. Masochism, on the other hand, which seemed to confuse Freud more than sadism, was explained as a tendency toward self-destructiveness. Even in their final form, however, Freud's theories have left us with many unanswered questions about the nature of sadomasochism.

Not all of the older ideas about sadomasochism were cast in such negative terms as those used by Krafft-Ebing and Freud. Havelock Ellis, for example, who recognized his own sadomasochistic interests, suggested that such desires might be traced to the play habits of sensitive children. He saw S&M as an outlet for atavistic impulses; one which left the individual more inclined toward tenderness in everyday life.

Perhaps the least negative approach to an explanation of S&M comes from the writings of Kinsey's colleague, Paul H. Gebhard. Dr. Gebhard, an anthropologist, believed sadomasochism to be a cultural phenomenon. That is, it has its origin in the norms and values of the larger social environment, rather than being an expression of idiosyncratic individual pathology. In his classic article on the subject, "Fetishism and Sadomasochism," Gebhard asserts the following:

> Sadomasochism is embedded in our culture since our culture operates on the basis of dominance-submission relationships, and aggression is socially valued. Even our gender relationships have been formulated in a framework conducive to sadomasochism: the male is supposed to be dominant and aggressive sexually and the female reluctant or submissive.

Gebhard continues his criticism, pointing a finger at media images that fuse sex and violence on the one hand, and perpetuate stereotypical sex roles on the other. Thus, Gebhard presents a purely cultural theory of the origins of sadomasochism. The problem with this theory, and with the others mentioned here, is that they only try to explain how S&M desires develop. They say nothing at all about how people become S&M practitioners, how they become involved with the S&M society, and how they come to form an S&M identity.

In order to explain these social-psychological events, we will be using the concept of "career." By "career" we mean a sequence of stages or steps along a path, with each career step suggesting a new level of involvement in leathersex and a new stage in the development of a leather identity. There are at least six such steps, which we have called "disenchantment," "depression," "curiosity," "attraction," "drifting," and "limiting."

DISENCHANTMENT

It is not unusual for younger, less experienced gay men to become somewhat disenchanted with the gay world a few years after coming out. This disenchantment may have any number of sources: the difficulty in forming a permanent relationship; frustrating experiences with over-possesive companions; the seeming insincerity, coldness, and shallowness of many bar games; or simple boredom with flashing disco lights, pretty faces, and excessive sex. This sense of disappointment with gay community night life is often intensified if hetero-culture norms (such as "monogamy-ideal" or "sex-means-love") are transplanted into the erotic reality of the homo-sexual male. These norms seldom work well in the context of all-male sexuality.

The most frequent complaint among disillusioned newcomers is that the average bar-going gay man is simply not "macho" enough to be attractive. The "straight" world conceptions of masculinity, usually ranging from the beer-drinking butch image to the overweight biker, often linger in the minds of those who are new to the gay scene. The more relaxed masculinity and manners of many gay men seems less erotic when compared with the hyper-masculine milieu of the straight world. Newcomers sense this disparity more deeply than other gay men, often leading them to a second step toward leathersex, a time of depression.

DEPRESSION

During the depression period, some gay men experience isolation anew — a second "closet." They often leave gay night life behind, returning to earlier days of loneliness and a fantasy sex life.

This depression may last from a few months to a few years, with different degrees of severity. Lasting periods of depression are typically marked by sexual outlets not traditionally part of the gay club and night life. Such outlets may include truck stop and tearoom encounters, adult bookstore and movie house pickups, sex ad liaisons, and adventures with hustlers.

Commonly, the age at which gay men enter this second closet, if they do at all, is the middle to late twenties, depending upon when involvement in the gay community first began. Further, most of those who experience a second closet eventually re-enter the gay world with more appropriate expectations; but some others do not. For some men, the second closet is a period of psychological preparation for another facet of the homosexual experience, the world of leather. This preparation involves movement to yet a third step, that of curiosity.

CURIOSITY

The gay man in his second closet, unlike the man in his first, has a working knowledge of the gay subculture. He knows the rules of interaction; where clubs, taverns, and organizations are located; and how he may participate. He is also wiser about his sexual orientation and his consequent position in society at large. Many of the anxieties he was forced to grow with, such as the belief that he must be the only homosexual in town, have since disappeared. In his second closet, he is aware of what he is missing.

The leather scene, however, like other minority elements of the gay community, may still be mysterious to him. It is likely that he knows only the stereotypes about S&M, as they may have been introduced to him by some of his first gay acquaintances. Such stereotypes of leathersex label it "emotionally distant," "sexually immature," "physically dangerous," and "preoccupied with hypermasculinity," all misguided perceptions of sadomasochism.

The stigma of exaggerated masculinity may lead some discouraged gay men to become curious about the S&M scene and to wonder whether a compatible partner might be found among the ranks of the leather clique.

Increasing curiosity often encourages a person to seek out more information about leathersex. Avenues of such information may include perusals through both pornographic and nonpornographic periodicals; questioning friends; weighing heresay, myths, and rumors; and visiting leather-oriented establishments. The latter may include out-of-town visits to S&M bath houses. As the search progresses, many individuals decide that leathersex is not what they want after all. They will find other alternatives for sexual expression, or drop out of intimate relations altogether. For many others who explore their S&M potential, an attraction may begin to develop.

ATTRACTION

As a man becomes attracted to leathersex, he may be laying the foundation upon which to construct an S&M self. That is, he may begin to believe that personal involvement in leathersex is at least plausible, and that he *could* be a participant if he wanted to. During the attraction stage, the perception that leathersex is within the bounds of one's erotic possibilities is crucial to the inception of an S&M identity. S&M activities must be conceivable before they can be seen as a part of the self.

This may also be a stage of growing excitement and anticipation about some future rendezvous with leathersex, when the individual might experience some physical and emotional contact. Social interaction often increases during this time, as does one's repository of knowledge about S&M. There may also be some contemplation about such rules-of-the-game as "limits," "signals," and other agreed upon safety devices. One discovers that leathermen have mutual respect for each other, and this information usually reduces fears of physical or emotional harm.

It is common for those men who become attracted to leathersex to be in their late twenties or early thirties, although this is far from a hard and fast rule. This stage involves a type of second coming out phase, when leather bars, baths, and perhaps bike organizations become a focal point of attention. Feelings of depression often diminish at this time, yielding to a growing drift into leathersex.

DRIFTING

Near the beginning of the drifting stage the novice commits himself to finding an S&M partner. He decides to experiment with leathersex. The search for an initial partner may be carried out in many ways, but probably the most common way is to increase visits to leather bars and baths. The diversity and variety of the leather crowd gives the person a chance to cruise for a compatible partner who is willing to train him.

Finding someone who will teach a beginner the ropes may not be so easy. One of the first discoveries a novice may make is that S&M experience is considered an asset among many leathermen; personality, youth, or good looks alone will not usually attract a mate. An initial encounter might therefore require an exchange of relative youth or good looks for senior "know how."

Leathersex requires by its nature a certain amount of acting ability. A successful (i.e., satisfying) encounter depends very much on the capacity of the participants to sustain each other's erotic fantasies. Inexperienced men are sometimes not aware of this unwritten rule, and seem interested only in their own sexual satisfaction. They have not yet fully appreciated the vital psychological link between their desires and those of their partner. This requirement of interdependence for psychosexual fulfillment is something better apprehended only after a number of S&M episodes have occurred. To experienced leathermen, rookies often appear unable to feign the appropriate leathersex attitudes in order to set aside their own needs and to satisfy the erotic requirements of their partner. This is why newcomers are so often viewed as selfish, both during and after leather scenarios.

Inexperience in developing and sustaining mutually satisfactory scenarios may also help to explain why the novice tends to prefer the role of the bottom. As slave, the beginner is able to enter S&M scenes more easily because he is supposedly led by his master into the various activities that make up the drama. His script is prescribed for him. After some period of drift in sexual slavery, the bottom usually decides that he too would like to lead. It is perhaps this decision, combined with learning the nuts-and-bolts of "what masters do," that allows the slave to begin taking the role of the top. The bottom-to-top path, as most leather enthusiasts know, is typical of the S&M career.

The period of drift is probably the longest period of all. It is actually a cluster of phases in which the leatherman makes a "new sense" of each activity in which he engages. It is a period during which previously uninteresting sexual behaviors gradually become a part of his erotic desires. As drift into sophisticated leather practices continues, the individual finds himself enjoying sexual practices once thought to be meaningless or silly.

During this drifting and sense-making process, a leather identity emerges. The person begins to see himself as a part of the S&M scene. He feels as though he is a member of a particular group of men. No longer a novice or a newcomer, he is more in control of the sexual situations in which he becomes involved. He is now ready for many more S&M encounters.

Drifting is often the step in a leather career in which new relationships with other gay men develop. The person may prefer a pattern of casual sex with a series of mates, or settle into a monogamous relationship. He may go through cycles of greater or lesser sexual interest and involvement. Whatever his preferences, he eventually reaches the final step of limiting.

LIMITING

A person enters the limiting stage when he experiments with one or more erotic acts and chooses not to make a new sense of them, those he perhaps wishes he had not tried. Instead of being able to assign feelings of pleasure to these behaviors, he experiences some anxiety. While drifting he is, of course, in a process of expanding his limits, not yet certain about the boundaries of his S&M tastes. During the limiting period, however, he practices leathersex with more or less full awareness of what he will and will not enjoy.

The leathermen who reach the limiting stage in their S&M careers are perhaps the most sexually satisfied (and satisfying) of all. They have defined the boundaries of their sexuality, and they are most likely to appreciate the needs and limits of others. With a fuller understanding of S&M, experienced leathermen often are better equipped to use good judgment during hot and heavy encounters.

The range of erotic variations in leathersex is probably greater than many gay people suspect. This makes limiting even more important in S&M. Failure to limit might prove unpleasant. Leather society has an elaborate system of spoken and unspoken social rules, dos and don'ts that govern the action of its members. Limiting underlies many of these rules.

Conclusions

The six-stage career framework used here does not apply to every sado-masochist. In fact, it probably fits well for only a very few. To suggest otherwise would be to disregard one of the most fascinating aspects of the leather world—the wide variations of actors and scripts. However, among many leathermen these steps are remarkably typical, representing the various stages that seem to be important in becoming a sadomasochist.

The S&M reality is sometimes thought to be a negative facet of the gay community, a thorn in the side of liberation. S&M is sometimes viewed as inconsistent with the ideology of the present generation of gay people, which holds that homosexuality is, and ought to be, the love of one's own sex in its pure, natural, and most beautiful form. Just as this view shuns playing daddy (pederasty), playing favors (prostitution), or playing lady (cross-dressing), it also refuses to sanction playing roles (sadomasochism). Sadomasochists not only voluntarily adopt roles, they overstate them, something gays often see as a heterosexist problem. Still, S&M is a topic about which most gay people are at least willing to talk. This is usually not true among heterosexuals. It is perhaps this relative degree of openness that explains why leathersex is practiced within a context of social rules and norms, and why it does not involve any real violence, coercion, or human abuse. Heterosexual culture, by contrast, does not readily tolerate open discussion about sadomasochism. Indeed, most heterosexuals probably do not know much about what it is, whether they harbor such feelings or not.

REFERENCES

Gebhard, Paul H. "Fetishism and Sadomasochism," pp. 71–80 in Jules H. Masserman, ed., *Dynamics of Deviant Sexuality,* New York: Grune and Stratton, 1969.

Krafft-Ebing, Richard von. *Psychopathia Sexualis* (Franklin S. Klaf, trans.), New York: Stein and Day, 1965.

Howard Smith and Cathy Cox

Dialogue with a Dominatrix

At the age of 19, an incredible dominatrix has taken center stage in New York's S&M netherworld. Making her living for the last two years from this controversial carnalmania, she's not exactly a bondage and domination beginner.

Originally, I came across Toni Rose during one of those open-to-the-public, Chateau 19, S&M soirees when, whip in hand, she walked into the crowded room, wearing a black cowboy hat, black leather mini-dress, and thigh-high, spike-heel boots, also black. Even in dangeroso duds, her face looked angelic. But through the course of the evening, as she teased, humiliated, and abused, I saw differently. Without seeming to try, she unquestionably captured scores of slaves' imaginations. Victim after victim told me that Mistress Rose was in a class by herself—"realer" in her sadism than any other mistress they had ever met. Portioning out pain in carefully calculated doses, she was oblivious to the unrelenting crowd of voyeurs constantly checking her out.

Seeing the cadre of submissives hover around her, like the revered Queen Bee, I wondered how such a young woman had gotten so deeply into her bizarre occupation. What thoughts seized her mind while she plied her trade? An interview was in order. Here are some revealing highlights about her unusual life:

Scenes: You started in the S&M scene when you were 17?

Toni: Yes. My mother, who went by the name Morgetta, was a professional dominatrix. I picked it up from her.

S: At what age did you become aware of what she was doing?

T: I was 10. We lived down South and she used to take me to the places where she worked and I'd sit and watch while she did things to men.

S: What did you think?

T: Well, she'd always tell me that she was punishing men because they deserved it.

S: But she didn't involve you in the scene.

T: No, no. I just sat there. I suppose it excited the men, too, knowing a child was watching all the activities.

S: What was the rest of your life like at that age?

T: Nothing really heavy. I just went to school, had my little boyfriends and everything. . . . I didn't have my own whips.

S: Did you ever act out your mother's routines on your friends?

T: Yes, as a matter of fact. Once I put on a little S&M show. The mother of the child that I was performing on got a little bit hysterical. She called my mother.

S: What happened?

T: I didn't play with her daughter anymore.

S: What did your friends think of you back then?

T: Oh Lord, they didn't know what to think. I'd wear these T-shirts that my mother handed out which said Morgetta the Wild One Lets It All Hang Out. But I wasn't worried about it; I just went on doing my thing. Actually, I had a typical teenage sex scene until I got into S&M two years ago.

S: Are there other kids in your family?

T: I have a half-brother, who was a deacon of the Baptist Church by the time he was 12.

S: How does your mother feel about you taking up the business?

T: She loves it; she really does.

S: Have the two of you ever done an S&M scene together?

T: No, once someone tried to book us but my mother didn't go for the idea. On the other hand, I would have been proud to share the stage with a dominatrix like her. She's wonderful at it.

S: What reasons do men give for seeing you?

T: A lot of the men who have sessions with me believe they should be disciplined for being chauvinistic. Since they've been sadistic toward women, they want a woman to be sadistic toward them. Some tell me they should be punished for no other reason than the fact that they were born; others say all men should be disciplined simply because women are superior.

S: Do you feel that way?

T: No, I feel men and women are equal.

S: So then, is this just a job to you?

T: No, being a dominatrix isn't *just* some job. I am very into what I do.

Instead of feeling that men are inferior, I believe they deserve to be disciplined and dominated for being so rude in the past to women. On another level, I feel like I'm acting as a form of therapist. Men come to see me and I do what they want. Then, after the session, they smile and walk out, ready to conquer their world again. A lot of the men who see me are important with heavy responsibilities for making a lot of difficult decisions. They come to me so that they can release some of the pressure and tension of having to be the one who's always in charge. With me they can finally be submissive. They get off on having someone else finally telling them what to do—sort of a reverse in roles.

S: What kind of men come to see you?

T: Basically, my slaves are upper-class men with families—the tweed-suit types. One guy, oh my god, he has so much money he brings his own very expensive equipment in a snake skin suitcase. He has an incredible collection of whips, some of them from Egypt.

S: What do you normally get for a session?

T: An hour usually costs $75.

S: And how do people get in touch with you?

T: I used to run my photo and an ad in *Screw* and, as soon as I get my new place together, I'll start publicly advertising again. Right now, though, I'm just seeing my regular following.

S: Do you ever have total novices call you?

T: Sure. Most of them of course, are usually very shy. They'll call seven times, or so, to make an appointment before they ever show up. Their session is basically just worshipping my body, getting verbally abused, a slight spanking, or dressing up as a transvestite. I start them off very mildly.

S: Do they always move on to the harder stuff?

T: Oh, no. With a lot of them, the fantasy is just bondage, the act of getting tied up.

S: Do they tell you what they want in advance?

T: Right, and before the appointment we work out a rough script, and then at the session I add my own improvisations.

S: Where did you study knots, in the Girl Scouts?

T: Yup. I was a Girl Scout. And I was in ROTC in high school and in the Drum and Bugle Corps.

S: Really?

T: Really.

S: What about the equipment you use?

T: I make my own cock whips, but I have a slave make my other leather goods for me.

S: What's a cock whip?

T: It's a small rawhide whip, about six- to eight-inches long that's used to spank the cock of slaves who are into penis torture.

S: What are some other common fetishes?

T: There's TV (transvestism), penis and nipple torture, golden showers, which involves urinating on someone, scat, which is shitting on someone, infantilism where the slave wants me to treat him like a baby. And then there are the popular fantasies, like my favorite, the Nazi interrogation where I come in with a little mini-Nazi outfit, including a swastika and my riding crop, and make a slave divulge the information. Or the nurse fantasy where the guy comes in as if he has an appointment in a doctor's office. I have these charts and just carry on from there—making him take off his clothes and then finally taking off my nurse's uniform and revealing all my black leather goods underneath. And then, of course, there is the foot fetish—a lot of men are hung up on women's feet.

S: Why do you think?

T: More than likely they used to watch their mother dress and got into the femininity of putting on the stocking or something like that. The foot is a very sensual part of the body.

S: What takes place with a foot fetish?

T: Well, one of my slaves likes to pretend he's the janitor. He vacuums the floor while I sit on the couch. When he's done, I tip the ashtray over with my toe and then he cleans the mess up and makes love to my foot, talking about the pink plumpness of my arch. Afterwards, he'll give me a hot soapy foot bath and a pedicure and that's how he achieves fulfillment.

S: He actually has an orgasm that way without having any genital contact?

T: Yes. In fact, I've even whipped guys and made them come even when they weren't hard.

S: Do you offer any special fantasies?

T: I love to encase a slave in Saran Wrap from his neck to his feet with the arms by his side so that he can't move. I call it "The Wrap." Then I give him a spanking with my hands. It's very effective because the plastic leaves the body real taut.

S: Are you always trying to come up with new ideas?

T: Yes, as a matter of fact currently I am interested in pulling off a kidnapping, not a real kidnapping, of course, but a staged fantasy, where I'd meet up with a slave who will be carrying an envelope of money. I'd pull up in a limousine and order him into the car. Then I'd take him away and tie him up. At a certain point, I'd release him and keep the ransom.

S: Since slaves pay you, they haven't really given you all the control, correct?

T: Maybe so, but the frightening part of it is that they *would* do whatever I say—anything at all. If I told them to sit on the stove while the burner was on, they would. I haven't asked anyone to do that, but I do have *that* much control over them.

S: How do you decide how far you'll go with a man?

T: Well, if they say heavy domination, then you know.

S: But at what point do you say, "No, I won't do this." For example, will you draw blood?

T: I have drawn blood, but the man wanted me to. He was into heavy dominance, and begged me to whip him until he bled, so, I did it. But, basically, bondage is what I prefer to get into, tying someone up and suspending him from the ceiling on a hoist. I'm not really into heavy pain. I'm more interested in the power of fear, making someone afraid. A lot of slaves get off on that.

S: Are you saying that part of the relationship that you develop with a slave is based on teasing, making them think that you would do something that you actually wouldn't do?

T: Exactly. It's like taking a match and putting it up against the body, but instead of burning anyone with it I just make the person afraid of the match. For some it's the fear of the whip, not the actual whipping, that gets them. They get off on what they think I'm going to do.

S: Do you ever refuse to do certain things?

T: Yes, I won't do scat, that's brown showers. Water sports, like urinating on someone, are all right. But I won't shit on a slave, or anyone for that matter. There are too many germs.

S: Did you do it once and it turned you off?

T: Yes, I became very mad at the slave and punished him for wanting it.

S: Do you ever see women?

T: Yes, I currently have two female slaves.

S: Are there any differences between a male and a female slave?

T: With a female slave, it's just more erotic and sensual in nature. A male is more oriented toward punishment. Personally, I've always enjoyed the scene of two women together.

S: Two women, meaning you as one of them?

T: Oh, yes. Or I'll have two slaves perform and just sit back on my pillows, smoke my cigarettes, and sip my drink while watching them carry on.

S: Do you ever get turned on when you're a dominatrix?

T: Oh yes, it's very erotic for me.

S: Do you ever reach climax?

T: Yes, I have.

S: Without genital contact?

T: Yes.

S: But what about falling in love? Have you ever really been involved with a person?

T: Yes, I really fell for this one foot-fetish friend of mine, who looks like Harry Reems, the porn star. Once when he was leaving, I tried to kiss him. But, I burst his whole fantasy wide open; I haven't seen him since.

S: Why do you think you fell for him?

T: He was so submissive. I guess I also knew that I couldn't have him. Then again, maybe it was because I really have a thing for Harry Reems. He looked like a younger version; that probably did it.

S: Do you ever have sex, genital or oral, with slaves?

T: No. I have private slaves that I call pets who service me and make me happy.

S: What's the difference between a slave and a pet?

T: Pets don't pay.

S: Does every slave get to be a pet?

T: No, when I feel a client has been disciplined enough to be a pet, then they get to do my bidding for me—only then.

S: Would every slave want to be your pet?

T: Oh yes, that would be like making it to the top of the ladder. For one thing they wouldn't have to pay anymore, and they'd get special treatment.

S: How many pets do you have right now?

T: Seven, three of them females. Each one has a certain function—I have a maid; I have someone who cleans out the fireplace; another cleans the bathroom, and then there's a slave, a male in a little apron, who is chained to the refrigerator. It's nice to have a man tied to the kitchen.

S: Sounds like every woman's dream. How long does someone get to remain your pet?

T: For as long as I want or until I am bored.

S: It's been said by professionals who have written books about sadists and masochists that most of these people switch from one role to the other. Is that true with you?

T: I'm absolutely dominant. I don't appreciate the switchables.

S: You don't have fantasies at all about being submissive?

T: No, I'd rather fight than switch.

S: What if Harry Reems himself called up and said, look. . .

T: Oh, well, for Harry Reems or for the Harry Reems lookalike . . . maybe.

S: In other words, if you really fell for someone.

T: Maybe so. Maybe it's love that makes you submissive at times. Actually, once it did happen to me. I was involved with a woman and the relationship kind of floated along until my domination left off and submission began. We were incredibly close. But it got to be too much; she had to move out.

S: Do you think everyone has some S&M in them?

T: Yes, at least slight tendencies. For example, when I tell people what I do, they always react by saying, "Well, I've never been into it, but I'd sure like to try it with you."

S: You talk freely to strangers about what you do?

T: Of course, I think it's amusing when people ask me what I do for a living. They seem to like it; they really do. I'll tell them I'm a dominatrix and if they don't know what a dominatrix is I'll say it's sort of like

Beardsley Impromptu Theatre. And if they say, "What's that?" I'll say, well, I whip men for a living. Then they ask me all about it and I tell them about foot fetishes, my T-shirts that say "I've Kissed the Toes of Mistress Rose," and my handmade "bondaids," bandaids that I stick onto the backside of every slave that I whip. A lot of these guys end up as my slaves. They trust me.

S: Where do you see it going for you in the future?

T: Having my slaves and my maids and my human candlesticks, I'm a pretty happy person. Maybe someday it would be nice to have a townhouse, a live-in maid to service me all the time.

S: So that's your ultimate goal . . . just making enough money to have a bigger scene?

T: If that happens, then it's all well and good. I wouldn't mind all the fame and glory of becoming the dominatrix of the century, but I enjoy myself as I am right now, you know, being a dominatrix and having my own seven pets.

Scenes would like to thank Burt Shulman for his assistance with this interview.

Juliette

Autobiography of a Dominatrix

It was 1968. Young people were claiming a new type of independence and completely shunning the customs and morals of the older generation. Everybody seemed to be getting involved and experimenting. I was only seventeen years old, restless, and curious about it all. I wanted to be involved and involved I got.

I had my bags packed for a year before I left for New York City. I left with a girl friend the day after our high school graduation ceremonies. I can still remember my mother driving us to the airport that morning, all the time warning me about the perils of the big city. But I just laughed at her, because what did she know about life anyhow? Besides, it would be different for me. I would have a good life, and I was a big girl now and could take care of myself. I had twelve hundred dollars in my pocket when we arrived. This was supposed to tide me over until I could find some type of employment. We stayed with a friend we had met that Easter when we came down to the city to spend the weekend. He was a photographer and an antique dealer and wanted to get my friend involved in modeling. She was a truly beautiful girl, the kind that you see on the cover of *Seventeen* magazine. Everybody made a fuss over her and told her how great she was. By the end of the month she was working as a photographic model and meeting just the right people. It was just like in a storybook. I, on the other hand, was always in her shadow. Nobody even noticed that I was alive. Besides, I was overweight and this made me even more despondent, unhappy, and extremely jealous. I wanted to be popular and have men notice me like they did her.

Specially written for this volume.

The nights were exciting in the city, and I was meeting people in clubs that I had only seen on the T.V. and heard on records. It was about this time that I really got involved in the whole drug subculture. It was through a woman that I met at a club one night. She was a groupie who would sleep with anybody who was in a group, or with any man for that matter. We got an apartment together on the city's Lower East Side right next to the Electric Circus and around the corner from the Fillmore East. My friend seemed to know about everything and she knew everyone in the Village. On Friday and Saturday nights her friends would come in from Brooklyn and the Bronx to go to the Circus but would first stop by our house and shoot up. We used to call them weekend junkies. These were people who would only get high once a week or so just for kicks. I had no say about what was going on in the apartment, it was like she had complete control over me. I just went along with anything she said.

She would always coax me to try dope. "I just want you to feel the rush," she would say to me "and if you sit still you won't get sick." So one night I finally consented. I can remember that night as if it were yesterday. I put out my right arm, closed my eyes and let the sweet juices of Miss Heroin flow into my veins. She was right. The rush was fantastic and I sat very still and didn't get sick. This was to be the beginning of a very long love affair with the White Lady. I started to shoot up pretty regularly then and my money was soon gone. But never fear because my friend was here. She knew two guys who would give us $25 apiece if we would just go to bed with them. I didn't want to do it, but once again she talked me into it. I found out that it wasn't all that bad. We took the money that we made and didn't pay the rent, but instead we spent it on getting high. We soon lost the apartment and went our separate ways.

I was alone with nowhere to go and no money in my pocket. For weeks I drifted from place to place and only rested when I could find an apartment to crash at. I was so scared and was getting sick from not eating and never resting. . . .Back out on the streets again, I met a man and we hooked up together and started selling heroin. The dope we had was good, and before you knew it we had a booming business and I had a habit as long as my arm—a dealer's habit. We made lots and lots of money and shot lots and lots of dope. I was secure once again. This sense of security didn't last for very long however, because after a few months of heavy dealing we finally got busted. The only thing left to do in order to survive and to keep a hole in my arm was to start turning tricks.

I really didn't know anything about the business at that time because I had only done it once before. But I was a trooper and quickly learned the ways of the ho' stroll.[1] I really didn't have any choice because I was now a bona fide junkie and had a dealer's habit besides. The area that I started on was E. 14th Street, the armpit of prostitution. Eighty percent of the girls who worked that area were junkies. Most of the tricks that were turned were done in cars—quick blow jobs. Home for me now had become the Valentine Hotel. This was the sort of place that girls turned tricks in and where welfare people and derelicts lived. The decor of the place wasn't anything you'd see in *Better Homes and Gardens* magazine. It smelled, but so did I. The people on the streets never bothered me much, because I always stayed to myself, trying to make myself invisible to the pimps and especially to the police. There was never any time to sleep because you had to find the money for your next fix. That was all that was important. The only time you got to relax was if you made a big sting.[2] Then you would just get a room and shoot up until the money was gone and you had to start the whole process all over again.

One night, while I was walking the streets looking for someone to pick up, I ran into this guy who told me that he was an ex-cop and asked me if I would be interested in working in a house with a Madam. I looked pretty dirty and grubby and couldn't understand what he wanted with me. He said if I wanted to, he would take me over that night to meet this woman, so I went. She lived in this beautiful apartment building with a doorman and the whole bit. We went inside, and I was introduced to a rather plump woman about 25 years old. She explained to me that her business was all done through a book with numbers that she had accumulated over the years and some that she had bought from a Madam who was going out of business and getting married. She said that the tricks started at an average of $25 and up. I would keep half of everything I made and half went to her for setting up the date. This sounded great and I wouldn't have to be on the streets any longer.

I went to work for her the next day and made about a hundred and fifty dollars. It was easy; all the appointments were set up for me, and the Johns[3] were all real nice. But unlike working on the streets, I had to learn to take my time with the Johns and to be more generous with my body. Everything was working out good and I had stopped shooting dope and was buying Methadone on the street so I could function better. But all this time I'm working, I'm thinking how I can get hold of that book and just make all the money for myself instead of giving her half. I took a lot of money from her but never got the book.

From there I went on to work at other houses that had a different system of getting their tricks. I started to work for a man and his wife who started the business so they could pay off old gambling debts. It was sort of an arrangement that he had made with the people that he owed the money to. This house was set up in a brownstone. They rented the whole place and used all three floors. There were four girls who worked at a time. There were two women there who just answered telephones, and one who would answer the door and introduce the available girls. They got their business by placing ads in *Screw* magazine. Each girl was given a fictitious name and an article was run every week in the paper about how luscious she was and what her specialties were. Specialities ranged from French, Greek, and TV sessions to bondage.[4] The sessions ran for about 40 minutes and that included anything you wanted for as many times as you wanted. The rooms were big and beautiful and with real wood-burning fireplaces in every room.

The first day I worked there I had on a halter top and a pair of hot pants. I thought for sure that this would certainly attract some attention. My first trick was a priest. He was a regular at this place and was easy to take care of, all he wanted was a blow job and ran out after it was over like a scared rabbit. I went back downstairs after I was finished and just sat and watched as everybody got picked except me. Then this very nice-looking man came in and chose me. We went upstairs and went through the preliminaries and then I asked him what type of session he wanted. He told me that he picked me because of the hot pants that I was wearing. He said that he had been in a Nazi concentration camp as a child and that a woman in charge there had worn shorts and high boots like the ones that I had on. He was a sort of servant to this woman and she would make him clean her boots. She would do this by making him sit in a chair and then take the heel of her boot and grind it into his crotch. He said that even as a child this used to arouse him and now it was something that he had to have done to him at least once a month. This was the first time I had ever encountered this type of freaky request. And so I stood over him while he laid on the floor and ground my feet into his crotch. Other than this, his sex life was quite normal according to him, but he just had an obsession with this particular act. Most of the sessions I had while working at this house were mostly straight, mainly because they had no type of equipment to work with. But the few men who did come in and ask for special sessions gave me my initial knowledge of sadomasochism.

I worked in this place for about six months until I got fired because I was falling asleep on the customers, and they started to complain to the management. I was turning an average of fifteen tricks a day. This meant that my takehome pay every night was about $300. As soon as I got out of work I would catch a cab, and go down and see the drug pusher.

When I left this place I knew that I couldn't work the streets anymore, it just wasn't the same. So I got myself a job at another house. This was a specialty house that dealt mostly in various kinds of S&M sessions. This house was set up in the ground apartment of a huge complex. All the sessions were $75 apiece. It was a wonderland for the man who had exotic tastes in sex. We had every type of device imaginable to make you as uncomfortable as we possibly could. There were, to mention a few: whips, paddles, cat-on-nine tails, chains, leather binders, leather blindfolds, handcuffs, rope, stiletto shoes, nurses' outfits, enemas, suspension equipment, nipple clippers, penis stretchers, dildos of every imaginable shape and size, and vibrators. It was also fun to make up your own types of tortures. It was incredible the things you could do with just a simple pair of tweezers and a candle stick. But not every man liked to be physically tortured. Some of these gentlemen just preferred to be verbally humiliated, or spanked with just your hand while you told them how naughty they were. But let us not forget the man who enjoys golden showers or to be defecated on. The average person might think that men who enjoy this type of perverted sex must be monsters. On the contrary, they were mostly professional people like lawyers, doctors, executives, or people in the arts. It wasn't bad working these kind of sessions. I mean, God, anything was better than flat-backing and having to be mauled and pulled at all day long. Besides, by this time I was pretty hardened and I enjoyed beating and humiliating men who had done the same to me. And when I got into a session I would put every ounce of strength I had into it. I hated all of these bastards: No matter how nice they were, they were still all just tricks to me, and disgusting. There was the fat man with club feet who would come to see me every week just so I could tell him how disgusting and repulsive he was, for which he always gave me a big tip. And there was a nice German gentleman who came to see me once a week to have his fanny beaten with a hair brush. He would take off all of his clothes and go hide in the bathroom and I would pretend I was his older sister and discovered him doing something naughty. He would act just like a small child and say, "I didn't do nothin'." I would pretend to get mad at him for lying to me, grab him and throw him over my knee and beat him with the brush until his whole ass was just one big red welt. This man also always gave me a good tip.

Men who are into things like role-playing usually pay very well when they can find a pro who's a good actress and who knows what she's doing. It's very important to be as realistic as possible. Sometimes they like you to dress up for these sessions. This was really popular with people who liked enemas. The whole thing of seeing a sadistic nurse in her little uniform while she makes a man take in all the water from a two-quart enema bag is just the biggest turn-on in the world for some people. Then there were the men who were leather worshippers and just adored seeing a woman dressed in a black leather jumpsuit and high heel leather boots. They would get very excited just touching the leather and loved to take their tongues and lick your boots all over. It's funny the way the most ridiculous things can turn some people on. Some people would want a session that they had never tried before just because it sounded like it might be exciting in their mind's eye. But once they actually do it, it's a whole other ball game. Sometimes, thinking about a perverted act can be much more exciting than the act itself.

We also advertised out of *Screw,* but we would put pictures of the girls in the ads. This place was in full swing for about eight months, at which time I managed the house and collected the money from the girls and paid them at the end of the night. One day, someone in one of the other apartments got wind that there was a house of ill repute in the building, and the whole neighborhood was in a panic. They had petitions that they were passing around the block for the people to sign to get us out of the building. They constantly harassed us and said that they were being attacked by the customers who came to see us. Well, we finally had to close the place down because it was impossible to work there any longer; so then everyone had to look for new employment. I looked through the trade papers and found an ad where they were looking for girls for a strictly outgoing service. I met a young man who had heard about what happened at the other place I was working at and he told me about this man who was looking for someone to run a house for him and to be his partner. I would not have to make any kind of investment, and the apartment and phones would be provided for me. He would be a silent partner and all he wanted was his share of the money every month. This seemed too good to be true. I told him the experience that I had and that I had owned several of my own houses before, which was a lie. But, damn, I had accumulated enough knowledge by now to run ten houses. He dropped off the keys to the apartment the next day; we moved in the house and prepared for the grand opening of "Cosmopolitan Playgirls."

We placed only one large ad in the paper. Basically, it stated that we were an outgoing service and would travel to any of the boroughs, including New Jersey, and, of course, that we specialized in discipline. Business was really slow for the first couple of weeks; there was only myself and another girl working, and one driver. The driver knew a woman who was a nurse and who was interested in working. I talked to her on the phone and we made a date for her to come down so I could interview her. She was super! She walked into the apartment wearing a full length mink coat with a studded dog collar around her neck, and she carried a whip made out of a horse's tail. When she took off her coat she had on a black leather halter top, shorts, and black leather boots with reinforced iron fronts for kicking better. She loved S&M not only for the money, but she also did it on her own time. When I told her that we were only charging $50 an hour she said that she refused to work for so little money, and I should have a starting price of at least $100 an hour plus the driver's fee. I told her that she was crazy, that there wasn't an ad in the paper that was charging over $65 now. She said that I could easily get that much money and got on the phone and set up my first $100 date. I learned that I could charge astronomical prices if I had the right girls, a good sales pitch, and, of course, tons of equipment.

The business started to grow, and before you knew it I had ten girls working for me, two phone girls, and five drivers. All the girls who were working for me had never worked in a house before. I had a college girl, a nurse, a housewife, a professional model, and a woman who worked in the kitchen of a famous hotel, all part-time working girls. These girls were not hardened by the streets or pimps and rather enjoyed what they did. The tricks loved it, and all the girls were beautiful and, most important, every one was happy and making big bucks. After the business got in full swing, we upped our prices for the S&M sessions and just had the straight sessions at $100. I completely stopped working now and just took care of the management part of the business. I felt like a queen, like I had finally made it. We started to entertain such people as foreign ambassadors, and my girls were escorts for many important business clients who wanted to entertain associates. The money was coming in like crazy and just as fast as it came in I spent it on drugs and clothes. My environment had changed and so had my standard of living, but I hadn't changed at all. I now had the opportunity to make something of myself and save some money, but I didn't. Even the girls were getting disgusted with me and started leaving. It finally ended with me getting arrested for promoting prostitution. I'll never know to this day how it happened, except that one of the girls who worked for me dropped a dime.[5] I left New York after that, got on a Methadone program, and came back home after eight long and hard years of hustling.

I'm drug-free now and physically okay, but I still yearn for the excitement of the business and that secure feeling I had when I was high. I don't know if I'll make it in your world but I've never tried so hard in my life. So I'm just gonna keep on truckin' and maybe I'll succeed, or maybe I'll die.

NOTES

1. "Ho' stroll" is the vicinity where prostitutes congregate to meet customers.
2. "Sting" refers to getting money by cheating someone.
3. Johns are the customers of prostitutes.
4. "French" refers to oral-genital sex; "Greek" is anal sex; "TV" is the term for transvestism; and "bondage" is the tying up of a person.
5. dropped a dime: called the police

SCENES
S&M INTERACTIONS

Introduction

This section opens with Thomas S. Weinberg's article, "Sadism and Maso-chism: Sociological Perspectives." Weinberg discusses some of the sub-cultural aspects of the heterosexual S&M world. This highly suggestive selection is valuable not so much for the answers it provides, but for the questions it raises. It represents a preliminary attempt to view sadomaso-chism as a theoretically approachable phenomenon, drawing upon frame analysis to bring out the germane features of the S&M scene. Frame analysis, developed by sociologist Erving Goffman, conceives of human interaction as being bounded or "framed" by social definitions that give the behavior a specific contextual meaning. The meaning of what is happening is shared, and a variety of "keys" are used to cue participants into what is "really going on." Frames not only define interaction, but they also control and restrict it as well. They set forth mutually agreed upon limits, which participants accept as inviolable. So, for example, what may appear to the uninitiated observer as a violent act may really be a theatrical and carefully controlled "performance" from the perspective of the participants. Thus, we find in this article what is perhaps the first attempt to frame S&M in the dramaturgical mode, a conceptualization originally alluded to by Gebhard.

Kamel and Weinberg illustrate the diversity in S&M and show that par-ticipation in this behavior is part of a social process by viewing involvement in sadomasochism as a "career." They adopt this perspective from Erving Goffman, who has noted that people who share similar "stigmas" tend to have much the same experiences and come to view themselves and others in similar ways. In the presentation of a number of S&M biographies and in their discussion, it is made clear that becoming a sadomasochist is to a large extent part of an interactive process. Those who have recognized their sado-masochistic feelings must seek out others who share their desires. Then they must learn how to construct and control S&M scenes. Through socialization, they learn specific norms and values. Other people, who have not previously recognized any sadomasochistic interests, become involved in S&M through a variety of relationships.

Pat Califia's essay, "A Secret Side of Lesbian Sexuality," is valuable in a number of ways. Like the Kamel "Leather Career" and "Leathersex" articles elsewhere in this collection, she focuses on a specific S&M subculture. In her discussion of the lesbian sadomasochistic world, Califia gives us an insider's first-hand account both of S&M interaction and of how a participant (in this case Califia herself) structures, defines, and feels about what is going on. In this sense, her article links both identities and scenes by illustrating how "frames" are constructed in the S&M world to serve the needs of individual S&Mers.

The last selection in this section, "Sadomasochism and Popular Western Culture" by Gerhard Falk and Thomas S. Weinberg, illustrates the ways in which S&M concerns go beyond specific erotic subcultures and are found within the recreational spheres in modern Western societies. In their paper, the writers point out that S&M as an erotic, consensual, and recreational behavior has existed for at least two centuries in England and in the United States. They discuss S&M clubs and erotic poetry and books in the eighteenth and nineteenth centuries. Falk and Weinberg pursue this theme into modern times by examining contemporary movies, literature, and music that contain explicit sadomasochistic themes.

Thomas S. Weinberg

Sadism and Masochism
Sociological Perspectives

Sadism and masochism are two varieties of sexual behavior of which
description and analysis have been largely lacking in the professional
literature. Sadomasochism has generally been described only by psychiatrists; consequently, the social aspects of this behavior have been almost
completely ignored. Sadomasochism has been of interest to the legal profes-
sion and the lay public only when some highly publicized crime with sadomasochistic overtones has occurred. Examples of these instances include the
infamous English "Moors" murders,[1] the sexual mutilation and killing of
William Velten in New Mexico in 1974,[2] and the so-called "trash bag
murders" which were recently uncovered in California.[3] Sociologists of
deviance have largely neglected sadomasochistic (S&M) behavior. Some recent basic texts in the sociology of sexual behavior do devote a few
paragraphs or pages to this behavior, [4,5,6] but their observations are neither
systematic nor theoretical. A recent paper[7] attempts a more systematic
overview of the S&M subculture, but it lacks any theoretical organization.
Journalists[8,9] have also examined the sadomasochistic subculture, but their
work, too, is largely descriptive and usually confined to reporting events at
an S&M organization such as the Till Eulenspiegel Society in New York
City.

Although attempts to theoretically organize and explain sadomasochism
as a social phenomenon have not been made by sociologists, sociological
literature and theory do provide a number of helpful starting points. There

Reprinted from: *The Bulletin of the American Academy of Psychiatry and the Law,* Vol. VI,
No. 3, 1978: 284-295. Reprinted by permission of the author.

is, for example, a large literature on subcultural deviance which might be explored. Frame analysis, role theory, interactionist, phenomenological, and ethnomethodological perspectives might be profitably used to gain some insight into the world of sadists and masochists. This paper represents a tentative attempt to apply some of the current theoretical perspectives in sociology to a study of the social organization of consensual sexual violence.

Our data include fully transcribed interviews with participants in the S&M scene, including "amateurs" and professional "dominatrixes," materials from S&M magazines, literature and flyers from sadomasochistic organizations, and so forth. The S&M world includes professional and non-professional segments and both "straight" and "gay" subworlds.[10] Members of this world, however, may not necessarily perceive themselves along these lines. There are blendings and blurrings and crossings over from one part of this world to another. Advertisers in S&M contact publications often make a point of their "flexibility," "versatility," or "bisexuality."

There are two central features of the sadomasochistic world. The first is that much of this behavior occurs within a subcultural context. This is not surprising, since by its very nature, participation in this behavior requires at least two individuals, and necessitates some degree of social organization in order to be consummated. It is, of course, not uncommon for individuals to engage in solitary autoerotic sadomasochism, sometimes with tragic results.[11] A second feature of the sadomasochistic world is that this social organization is "framed"[12] in terms of fantasy, as a kind of theatrical production. Fantasy and theatricality are reflected, for example, in the roles available to players, their relations to one another, the kinds of scenes that are enacted, and the argot of the group.

THE S&M SUBCULTURE

Deviant subcultures form, according to Albert K. Cohen,[13] when individuals with common problems of adjustment come into communicative interaction with one another. The subculture, as a system of beliefs and values generated through this interaction, serves to help the individuals solve these problems. Although Cohen's work was concerned with delinquent youths, his ideas are applicable to other sorts of subcultures. People with sadomasochistic interests, like individuals with other nonmodal desires such as gays,[14] often recognize these needs quite early but are unable to act upon them, for they do not know that a world of their "own"[15] exists. They often feel isolated and "sick." Often their exposure to other sadists and masochists is fortuitous, as illustrated in the following conversation between an interviewer (I) and a respondent (R):

I: Okay, you were going to talk a little about S&M.
R: Yeah, I'm not really sure where to start. I've found I really enjoyed

it and always had fantasies about it. It's really good. What are some of the things you'd like to know about?

I: Well, for example, how did you first start thinking that you were interested in S&M and how did you eventually act out on it and so on?

R: Okay. Well, my fantasies, ever since early childhood, have always been masochistic. . . . And then, when I was developing a gay identity, my fantasies changed only a little. And I never really acted upon it, until I came onto somebody in (city) who was a sadist. And he was really an interesting person. He opened up a very fancy restaurant. . . . There's a gay community council in (city), and they held some of their meetings over in his restaurant. And I decided that I wanted to attend one . . . and also the restaurant manager was there and we just got to talking, you know. . . . And after everybody left, he just started talking to me and he just kind of closed off a part of the restaurant, and we just started having sex there and then we went into his office and more over there and then we went down to his room where he seemed to store dishes and stuff, it was completely closed off, and it got real heavy in there. And he treated me really special, I thought, giving me free food after that and giving me a ride home with somebody else. But after that I didn't see him because some of his friends seemed to have nicknames like "Godfather" and so forth.

I: Did you get into an S&M scene with him then?

R: Right.

I: What did you do? Did he tie you up? Did he initiate it or did you or what?

R: He did.

I: What did he do?

R: He didn't have any equipment or anything. There was a lot of slapping and he wanted me to masturbate in front of him and he wanted me to talk to his cock.

I: And then what happened? You said you didn't see him again?

R: Right. Afterwards, I really felt kind of elated and kind of like laughing and he said, "You're amazing!" Like he was completely flabbergasted by it.

I: Why, because you enjoyed it?

R: Yeah. I think that was it.

Other respondents met people interested in S&M through already established sadomasochistic organizations:

I: Can you tell me about (your first sadomasochistic act) and how it happened and so on?

R: Well, there's this place in New York called the Eulenspiegel Society.

I don't know whether you ever heard of it; it's kind of a place where all people, they call it sexual minority people, go, people with sado-masochistic behavior or gay people go there, straight people, bisexuals, some transvestites, a kind of real liberal place. And I met this guy there and he said he was interested in getting together in this act, this sadomasochistic thing. And I said, "Yeah, I'd like to try it." And, we went to his house, apartment in New York and I've always had fantasies around that area . . . but with this guy, I didn't get into it at all. I mean, you know, the fact of being tied up and getting hit with a belt. I just, I don't know, I thought I could get into it, but once it happened I just didn't get into it at all. I didn't like being fucked up the ass either. It hurt me.

I: Did you reciprocate? Did you do it to him?

R: No.

Some people discover the S&M world through other, related, deviant worlds. A professional dominatrix, for example, told the researcher that she had learned about sadomasochism through contacts with customers in a brothel:

I: How did you decide that you were going to specialize in S&M?

R: Well, I decided that because when I went into the houses to work I saw that that entailed more money. And it was interesting to me. Like, the first time I ever did it, like I took over the house and I was shooting so much drug, I was spending so much money on drug, I would be up one minute and I'd be back down on the streets the next minute. Then I'd fall into something else. And I was working in this house. The house was a very good house. This is how I first found out about *Screw* magazine and one day a guy came in and he needed somebody to do a dominance session with him. And I didn't know what to do. And one of the girls just said to me, "Well, here's some material," and told me what to do and I went up there and I took it from there and it was just something that came naturally to me.

I: What did he want you to do, do you remember?

R: It was a bondage session and a verbal humiliation session with whips.

I: What do you do during verbal humiliation sessions?

R: Well, you know, some guys just don't like anything else except to be verbally humiliated. You tell them that they're disgusting, you know, "You dirty son of a bitch." And, "You're this. And you're a pervert and look how ugly you are." All kinds of the worst things that you can think about somebody just to verbally humiliate them. You know, like maybe stand on their heads. Or stand on them and you're talking to them and just make them feel as low as you can.

You know, having them on the ground. Just stepping on somebody's head like that. People pay for it.

The other side of the professional S&M scene is reported by a man whose first sadomasochistic acts were with a prostitute:

R: This is a hangup (I had) with girls, because what I really was into was kind of a sadomasochistic thing, you know, and when I was young I really felt I could never talk to any girls about that. But then when I tried a few sexual acts with prostitutes and that, in that way, it was kind of enjoyable although there was no intercourse because it was more money. And so it was just kind of a scene with just masturbation.
I: And how did you feel about these experiences?
R: I really enjoyed them, but I felt guilty about it. Deep inside there was a lot of guilt. But I really enjoyed it.
I: Why did you go to the prostitutes, then?
R: Why?
I: Yeah.
R: I don't know. I guess just because I figured that a girl wouldn't. I don't know, a regular girl would be kind of turned off by, you know, fantasy called "abnormal" or "deviant."

Novices in sadomasochism may also attempt to make contacts through S&M magazines, sometimes advertising themselves as beginners, "New and into bondage," "New to these adventures but not turned off," and so forth.

Once subcultures are formed, they provide their members with techniques for engaging in certain kinds of behavior and with ideologies, "motives, drives, rationalizations, and attitudes"[16] that serve to normalize and even to elevate the individual's needs and behavior. In the case of S&M, techniques are taught not only through personal contact, but through letters and stories appearing in sadomasochistic publications. Some advertisers in contact magazines, in fact, offer to "train" and "dominate" respondents by mail. Numerous companies produce and advertise an endless variety of devices, costumes, and paraphernalia used in the "training" of S&M devotees.

The development of apologias, attitudes, and ideologies supportive of S&M appears to be more important than the dissemination of specific techniques for restraining people and inducing pain and discomfort. Statements of sadomasochistic organizations serve to justify and celebrate the activities of their members. For example, a Eulenspiegel flyer says:

What *is* S&M? Does the phrase conjure up vague visions of DeSade or Torquemada, or perhaps at best *The Story of O*? The subject has always been cloaked in fear and speculation, largely because of the shroud of ignorance born of traditional sex taboos.

The *Eulenspiegel Society* is an organization devoted to shedding light and joy on this neglected area of sexual fulfillment. Eulenspiegel is not in any sense a sex club or swingers' organization, but a discussion and consciousness-raising group that explores the cultural and psychological nature of *sexual dominance and submission,* sadism and masochism. It is the aim of this organization to promote better understanding and self-awareness of these drives so that they may be enjoyed as a part of a full sex life, rather than set aside out of fear or guilt.

Malibu Publications, which publishes the magazine *Amazon,* displays a similar rationale for sadomasochistic behavior in a flyer advertising their magazine:

As the name indicates this is a contact magaziner devoted exclusively to devotees of S&M/B&D*. It was launched just over a year ago in context with the philosophy that inasmuch as every human being harbors masochistic and/or sadistic tendencies, why not bring S&M/B&D out of the "closet" by tastefully presenting the subject as the normal sexual indulgence it really is. *Amazon* has achieved this! It provides the average person with a publication that reveals S&M/B&D as a normal form of sexual activity and alleviates any feelings of guilt and/or perversion arising from long held misconceptions.

These statements fall into the general category of what have been called "accounts," "linguistic device(s) employed whenever an action is subjected to valuative inquiry."[17] More specifically, accounts are statements "made by a social actor to explain unanticipated or untoward behavior. . . . An account is not called for when people engage in routine, common-sense behavior in a cultural environment that recognizes that behavior as such."[17] The kinds of accounts presented here are illustrative of what Scott and Lyman call "justifications." "Justifications are accounts in which one accepts responsibility for the act in question, but denies the pejorative quality associated with it."[17] In particular, one type of justification explicitly used in these apologias, is a device that Scott and Lyman term "self-fulfillment."[17] That is, the writers of these statements do not simply normalize sadomasochistic behavior for the initiated; instead, they attempt to enlighten outsiders about the "joys" of this behavior. Thus, the importance of these

---

*B&D" is Bondage and Discipline, which refers to controlling another person's behavior through physical restraints or bonds, or by verbal commands. Various punishments may be used to gain compliance. —*Eds.*

accounts is that they are not merely concocted by individual, isolated actors. They are, instead, socially produced, taught, reinforced, and continually reaffirmed by members of a given subculture or group. The group thereby does for the individual what he cannot do for himself. It provides him with external justifications for his desires and behavior. In a word, the subculture normalizes his orientation for him. Some of these accounts, more accurately, are "techniques of neutralization," similar in function and often in tone to those produced by gangs of delinquent youths.[18]

These sorts of apologias represent what Abraham Kaplan has called "reconstructed logic," in contrast with what he terms "logic-in-use."[19] Reconstructed logic is an *ex post facto* idealization rather than an accurate description of participants' motives as ongoingly displayed in actual S&M situations (logic-in-use). Compare, for example, the Eulenspiegel statement with journalistic descriptions of actual Eulenspiegel meetings and events,[8,9] or, for instance, with the statement of one participant, a professional dominatrix:

> Well, eventually I just, they were just business to me. I really didn't care for them at all. They were just money. It was just like getting in there and getting out of there. It was just a business, that's all. I hated them, especially when I got into the S&M thing, you know. Then I took out all my frustrations on them. I was very brutal.

FANTASY AND THE THEATRICAL FRAME

It is impossible to attempt to develop an understanding of the sadomasochistic subculture without examining the place of fantasy and theatricality in this world. The S&M scene is a fantasy world and can be most effectively understood in that light. Here we can profitably draw from the insights of Erving Goffman, especially with reference to his work on frame analysis.[12] Frameworks, according to Goffman, are perspectives or "schemata of interpretation," which, when applied by an individual to events, render "what would otherwise be a meaningless aspect of the scene into something that is meaningful . . . each primary framework allows its user to locate, perceive, identify and label a seemingly infinite number of concrete occurrences defined in its terms."[16] The kinds of frameworks with which we are concerned here are social frameworks. The theater is an example of one sort of social frame. Goffman notes that the primary frameworks of a particular social group are a central element of its culture.[12] These frameworks are embedded within the language of the group.[17] The language itself provides rules for their application within specific contexts, as well as defining particular roles, identities, and relationships within these contexts. The special argot of S&M works in this way.

Related to Goffman's discussion of frameworks is his concept of "keys" and "keying." A "key," according to Goffman is "the set of conventions by which a given activity, one already meaningful in terms of some primary framework, is transformed into something patterned on this activity but seen by the participants to be something quite else. The process of transcription can be called keying."[12] An example of keying would be action that appears to be fighting but has been transformed into play by the "combatants." Participants in the activity are consciously aware of the systematic alteration that is going on.

S&M activity appears to fall within what Goffman calls the "theatrical frame." Within this frame, various sorts of keyings are used by the participants: those which transform what might appear to an outsider to be violence into make-believe or a kind of play-like behavior, those which set limits, those which affect role switchings and the dominance order, and so on. An important aspect of any dramatic scripting, such as those which occur during a sadomasochistic episode, is that unlike the situation in the real, everyday world where a certain degree of uncertainty obtains, participants in this activity have the opportunity to "'play the world backwards,' that is, to arrange now for some things to work out later that ordinarily would be out of anyone's control and a matter of fate or chance." "In the case of make-believe," as Goffman puts it, "the individual can arrange to script what is to come, unwinding his own reel."[12] This is exactly what occurs in the S&M world. Participants interact within a particular (theatrical) frame, collaboratively setting specific limits to the scene. This limit setting is critical, as a respondent indicates:

> Usually, sometimes, when you have a new client, what I used to do was I used to sit down and I would talk to them first and find out exactly what they wanted. Because sometimes you can get into a session with somebody and get very brutal and that's not what they want. There's heavy dominance and there's light dominance and there's play acting, roles, all different kinds. So the best thing to do is to sit down and talk to somebody first, initially.

Devotees of S&M frequently indicate that it is the masochist who controls the interaction in a sadomasochistic episode. That is, he sets the limits by keying this activity as make-believe, something which is to be understood as not the "real thing." A male masochist, who defines himself as "bisexual," explains how he works out limits with his partner:

I: Someone tells me that in an S&M situation it's really the masochist who has all the control.

R: Uh huh.

I: Is that true?

R: Could be. I just read in (publication) that there's maybe no such difference as between passive and aggressive partners. That you can never be entirely passive or aggressive. . . . And, if I didn't want him to do something, I'd let him know. And he'd have to stop right there, because there's also, like, limits.

I: Is there a kind of understanding between S&M people, that you set out limits? You set these limits out before, or . . . ?

R: Before. Before each act. He liked to press me to do heavier and heavier things. But, uh, you definitely have to have a limit, before you go further. So, if I don't like it, you're not going to go on.

I: Are there certain things that you don't do?

R: Um huh. Yes.

I: Like what?

R: I really don't like being pissed on. Even though there's actually no pain involved. And, he wanted to stick pins in me. But he just gets near me with a pin and I jump ten feet.

An interesting phenomenon in the sadomasochistic world is what appears to be an overrepresentation of "dominant" women and "submissive" men. In a content analysis of two issues each of *Latent Image* and *Amazon,* popular S&M contact publications, the preferences (either "dominant" or "aggressive," or "submissive" or "passive") of advertisers who indicated an orientation were distributed as shown in Table 1.

Table I.

Self-Characterizations as "Dominant" or "Submissive" by Advertisers in S&M Contact Magazines

Magazine, Issue	Males N=201		Females N=480		Couples N=93		
	Dominant	Submissive	Dominant	Submissive	Both Dominant	Female Dominant/ Male Submissive	Male Dominant/ Female Submissive	Both Submissive
Latent Image, No. 11	8	27	39	5	2	9	6	2
Latent Image, No. 12	16	14	46	3	3	3	9	2
Amazon, No. 4	24	45	105	28	8	1	6	3
Amazon, No. 6	23	44	207	47	16	5	13	5
TOTAL	71	130	397	83	29	18	34	12

In the large proportion of cases, "submissive" women sought other women or couples. This was also true for couples in which the woman was the submissive partner. Some of the submissive women who advertised appear to really be half of a couple. In any event, it does not seem to be the case that "submissive" women seek out dominant men. As a recent text in "sex and human life" observes, "it is commonly the case that sadistic men cannot find a masochistic female partner."[6]

The presence of high proportions of dominant women and submissive men in a society in which men are supposed to be aggressive and women are defined as passive presents an interesting paradox which may be resolved by referring to the theatrical frame. Goffman observes that "frequent role switching occurs during play, resulting in a mixing up of the dominance order found among the players during occasions of literal activity."[12] Within a fantasy scene, traditional sex roles may be reversed without threatening the participants, if it is defined as "just make-believe." Roles are reversed, however, only in the sense that an individual who is "really" an adult male finds himself subservient to another who is "really" a female. But since the interactants are frequently acting out roles different from the ones which they "normally" occupy, very often the dominance order of the "real world" is sustained. That is, in the "real" world, some people (e.g., adults) have rights over others (e.g., children) where such rights include the administration of certain forms of corporal punishment, violence, and the like. Traditionally, males have such rights over females, hence, women's complaints at being "treated like children," and so forth. In a recent paper, for example, West and Zimmerman[20] find that there are "striking similarities between the pattern of interruptions in male-female inter-changes and those observed in the adult-child transactions" and interpret this to mean that "females have an analogous status to children in certain conversational situations (which) implies that the female has restricted rights to speak and may be ignored or interrupted at will."[20]

Much S&M activity follows general social-organizational patternings, so that when the relations are "reversed" (e.g., when the man gets beaten, degraded, etc.) metaphors like "governess"/"child," "mistress"/"slave," "teacher"/"pupil," and so forth are used to invoke a conventional patterning anyway. A dominatrix, when asked why she thought men had developed their particular interests, answered in terms of their childhood back-grounds, and pointed out that they often took child-like roles within the S&M interaction:

I: Have you ever tried to figure out why some of these people are into some of the things they're into?

R: Well, I didn't have to figure it out. I've asked them. A lot of them have talked to me about it. A lot of it stems from the way their mothers were, experiences they've had in childhood. A lot of it stems from, you know, things that have happened to them when they were kids. Something that impressed them when they were a child and it stayed with them for the rest of their lives. I had one guy that, I guess, his mother was on his back all the time. Another guy used to watch the spankings, and another guy that used to come in and I used to have to play his big sister and I'd stand in the bathroom while he would take something of mine, pretending that he was taking it out of the drawer and I'd have to come in and say to him, "What are you doing?" you know, and we'd go through the whole act. . . . I used to have a guy that used to come in, he used to like to put on diapers and play like you're a baby and you're supposed to pee on yourself or in a diaper, and things like that.

Some males who take the submissive role do so only when they are dressed as women. Others pretend to be dogs, horses, or other animals. S&M contact magazines are filled with ads from male transvestites and others who wish to participate in sadomasochistic activities in roles other than that of adult male, and from women who sustain these kinds of fantasies:

GODDESS ADRENA COMMANDS all humble & obedient servants to beg for application into her male DOG TRAINING classes. Beg to be my lap dog douche bag mouth & crawl beneath me always!

All bad boys int. in spanking, B&D, S&M, female domination or enemas write to Queen Linda, Glendale.

Well trained Dominant and exotic TV arranging for "Dude" ranch with fully equipped stables, dungeon, leather garments, etc. All dominant fems invited to participate. Male "Studs" must qualify through series of private training sessions. For further details & photos, write. San Francisco.

White male, 30, Bi-sexual, wishes to meet attractive, dominant woman or T.V. Couples OK if she is dominant. Dress me in frilly, silky, women's things and I will be your FR. maid or sisterly companion. Also enjoy leather & rubber. Lasting relationship possible. No professionals. Send photo and phone. Can & will travel, particularly to the N.E.

Men who are submissive would appear to be able to reconcile these needs with the societal pressures on males to be active, dominant, and superordinate to women by donning a special role within an S&M episode. Thus, it is the actor as a "child" ("slave," "female maid," "dog," etc.) who is being beaten, degraded, humiliated, and so forth, and not the person in his "actual social identity"[15] as an adult male. By taking a role which is not "really" his "own," the individual reinforces the definition of the situation as "play," "make-believe," "fantasy," and the like. This enables him to segregate the S&M situation from his everyday life. Professional prostitutes and dominatrixes often point out the apparent ease and rapidity with which clients can slip in and out of these roles.[21] A good deal of this has to do with keying of the activity. Specialized argot and terminology serves to cue the activity in and out for the participant. Fantasies, of course, are expressed in terms of this language, as is apparent from some of the contact ads presented above. It is important to note that fantasies are not unique, private, and idiosyncratic, but instead, involve *culturally general* resources – typifications of persons, of typical actions and situations, and so forth. Fantasies are part of the culture.

SUMMARY AND CONCLUSIONS

This paper represents an initial attempt to provide a theoretical structure for the sociological study of sadomasochism. Sadomasochistic behavior, like human behavior in general, is most fully understood within a social context. To understand "what is going on" within an S&M episode, one must know something about the culture of the group and how it defines and categorizes people and behavior. This is where frame analysis is helpful. Frames are central components of the culture of the group, through which its members interpret the world. To a great extent the frame itself is structured by the language of the group, which serves to explain to its members what is happening and to justify their desires, motives, and behavior. Frames tell people what is and what is not proper, acceptable, and possible within their world. They define and categorize for their members situations, settings, scenes, identities, roles, and relationships.

When people join sadomasochistic groups, or any other kind of group, they are taught not only frames, but also the conceptual tools or "keys" for defining, applying, transforming, and limiting them.

Frame analysis helps make sense of findings that might otherwise be difficult to explain. For example, the apparently puzzling existence in the S&M subculture of "dominant" women and "submissive" men when the larger society to which these individuals also belong prescribes aggressiveness for males and passivity for females may be explained in terms of make-believe, fantasy, and the theatrical frame. Lack of generalization into the larger world of roles and relationships developed within the sadomasochistic subworld is explained in terms of how behavior is "keyed."

A number of areas that have not been fully developed here could be profitably explored. For example, although we have attended to the structuring and limiting of S&M frames, we have not explored misframings, miskeyings, breaking frame, and other errors and their consequences for interactants. Hollander,[22] for instance, provides an example in which an S&M episode was miskeyed with disastrous results. Another issue for further exploration involves the ways in which the language of S&M structures the relations between participants in that world by building in notions of activity and passivity and tying these to particular roles in the interaction. The specific identities of people as "dominant" or "submissive," the ways in which they arrive at a recognition of these self-identities, and the stability of these orientations await investigation.*

NOTE

* A number of these questions are addressed by other essays in this collection. For example, Andreas Spengler discusses sadomasochistic role preferences and self-acceptance, G. W. Levi Kamel develops a theoretical structure for analyzing the acquisition of a "leatherman" self-identity among homosexuals, and Kamel and Weinberg explore the development and practice of sadomasochistic identities as an interactive process in "Diversity in Sadomasochism: Four S&M Careers." In this essay they give examples of the ways in which identities such as "dominant" and "submissive" evolve and are modified by the needs of one's partners. —*Eds.*

REFERENCES

1. The trial begins. *Newsweek* 67:34, 2 May, 1966.
2. Footlick J. K., Smith S.: Did the bikers do it? *Newsweek* 85:63-64, 17 Feb., 1975.
3. 2 homosexuals quizzed in 43 killings. *Buffalo Courier-Express:* 7, 4 Jul., 1977.
4. Gagnon J: *Human Sexualities.* Glenview, Ill.: Scott, Foresman and Company, 1977.
5. DeLora J. S., Warren CAB: *Understanding Sexual Interaction.* Boston: Houghton Mifflin Company, 1977.
6. Pengelley E. T.: *Sex and Human Life,* 2nd edition. Menlo Park, Calif.: Addison-Wesley Publishing Company, 1978.
7. Weinberg T. S., Falk G: Sadists and masochists: The social organization of sexual violence. Read before the Annual Meeting of the Society for the Study of Social Problems, San Francisco, Calif., 1978.
8. Coburn J.: S&M, *New Times* 8:43, 45-50, 4 Feb., 1977.
9. Halpern B.: Spanks for the memory. *Screw* 420: 4-7, 21 Mar., 1977.
10. Homosexuality: Gays on the march. *Time* 106: 32-37, 43, 8 Sep., 1975.

11. Dietz P. E.: Kotzwarraism: Sexual induction of cerebral hypoxia. (Unpublished manuscript.) Medical Criminology Research Center, McLean Hospital, 1978.
12. Goffman E.: *Frame Analysis.* Cambridge, Mass.: Harvard University Press, 1974.
13. Cohen A. K.: *Delinquent Boys: The Culture of the Gang.* Glencoe, Ill.: The Free Press, 1955.
14. Weinberg T. S.: Becoming Homosexual: Self-discovery, Self-identity, and Self-maintenance. (Unpublished doctoral dissertation.) The University of Connecticut, 1976.
15. Goffman E.: *Stigma: Notes on the Management of Spoiled Identity.* Englewood Cliffs, N. J.: Prentice-Hall, 1963.
16. Sutherland E. H., Cressey D. R.: *Principles of Criminology,* 6th edition. New York: J. B. Lippincott Company, 1960.
17. Scott M. B., Lyman S. M.: Accounts. *Am Sociological Rev* 33: 46-62, 1968.
18. Sykes, G., Matza D.: Techniques of neutralization: A theory of delinquency. *Am Sociological Rev* 22: 664-670, 1957.
19. Kaplan A.: *The Conduct of Inquiry.* San Francisco: Chandler Publishing Company, 1964.
20. West C., Zimmerman D. H.: Women's place in everyday talk: Reflections on parent-child interaction. *Social Problems* 24: 521-529, 1977.
21. von Cleef M.: *The House of Pain.* Secaucus, N. J.: Lyle Stuart, 1971.
22. Hollander S.: *The Happy Hooker.* New York: Dell, 1972.

G. W. Levi Kamel and Thomas S. Weinberg

Diversity in Sadomasochism
Four S&M Careers

The S&M world is a diverse subculture. Most probably it would not be inaccurate to say that there are a number of different S&M subcultures, or, perhaps, sub-subcultures. There are variations not only in terms of basic sexual orientations such as heterosexual and homosexual with many possibilities for blendings and crossings over, but there are also individuals and, consequently, social groups with tastes for various kinds of costumes and behaviors. There are, for instance, numerous gay leather and motorcycle clubs. There is allegedly a loose confederation of people with a fancy for "fist fucking" (The Fist Fuckers of America).[1] People who are "into" transvestism, enemas, urination ("golden showers" or "watersports"), defecation ("scat" or "brown showers"), whips, bondage, and the like can all find not only partners, but also newsletters, magazines, and clubs catering to their specific preferences.

The variety of sadomasochistic identities and behaviors makes the study of S&M both fascinating and challenging. S&M "careers"[2] can be studied as a social as well as a psychological phenomenon. That is, instead of making the individual as "patient" the sole focus of interest, as is done traditionally in clinical case studies, instead we can treat the individual as a *social actor* and examine his behavior from *his* perspective. We are especially interested in his definitions of situations, the ways in which he applies *socially acquired* meanings to situations and learns to make sense of what is going on through a process, of socialization to sadomasochism. Our focus here is very definitely on social interaction and the ways in which meanings are learned and shared as much as it is on the individual actor.

Specially written for this volume.

113

The following examples illustrate not only the endless varieties of career paths along which S&Mers travel, but they also point out the importance of other persons in teaching both behaviors and attitudes toward sadomasochism as a form of erotic expression. The nature of S&M as a collaborative event is obvious in all of these histories. For example, we can see how Jeanie is socialized by Daniel and the ways in which she has learned to accommodate herself to his needs. She has even come to define sadomasochist acts as pleasurable and erotically stimulating. Glen's career illustrates how an individual's perceptions and goals may change as a result of the learning experiences he has had with other S&M devotees. It also shows how S&M couples can segregate their sadomasochistic behavior from other areas of their relationship. Robbie's story points out the importance of mutual respect and affection for people involved in ongoing S&M relationships. Implicit in his history is that there are norms governing sadomasochistic interaction and that control is shared by both partners. Vito has not yet settled upon a relatively fixed sexual identity. We can see in his history the dynamic nature of S&M careers through the ways in which he tries to make sense of his feelings by experimenting with female prostitutes and male sexual partners.

DANIEL AND JEANIE: AN S&M RELATIONSHIP

Sadomasochism is perhaps best understood as an interactive phenomenon. It is above all a cognitive event that emerges as sadist and masochist confront each other. One way to understand S&M, therefore, is to take a look at relationships that are based heavily on the extremes in dominance and submission. Daniel, twenty-seven, and Jeanie, twenty-six, are one couple who practice sadomasochism. Married three years, Daniel and Jeanie have formed a strong S&M bond, which permeates their sexual life and their everyday activities. Their relationship began at a relatively early period in their lives, when Daniel was a sophomore in high school. A brief profile of Daniel and Jeanie as individuals is instructive before describing their life together.

Daniel has been interested in sadomasochism since he can remember. As a child, his daydreams took him on a number of mental excursions into masochism. He describes one of them:

I used to fantasize things like getting cornered by a bunch of girls on the playground and getting peed on just for fun. Sometimes I would think about getting tied up by them first. I was about twelve or fourteen then. . . . Oh yes, I would get erections with those thoughts, but I can't say how the thoughts started with me.

Later, Daniel recalls, his masochistic fantasies became more sexually explicit in nature. With remarkable clarity and detail, Daniel remembers,

> I would think about being tortured by two tall black women. I'd be in their apartment in the ghetto and they would accuse me of stealing their money. I took the money from their purses. They were dressed a little differently each time I thought of them, but always they had leather straps under their clothes, high heeled black boots, and steel toes. Usually I thought about them whipping me. They would strip me and torture my cock. They would sit on me and force me to perform oral sex on them. Just before the session was over they would give me permission to jack off.

It is often the case among male heterosexual sadomasochists that transvestic activities hold some erotic meaning. The meaning may be trans-sexual—the desire actually to be female—or it may signify humiliation, an important feeling for most masochists. In the latter situation, cross-dressing activities are fetishistic. That is, they involve sexual foreplay and orgasm. Daniel is no exception. Dressing at least partly in female attire has been a part of his erotic adventures since puberty. Beginning at the age of twelve or so, and until his late teens, Daniel used many of his mother's clothes for masturbation. Articles such as shoes, panties, brassieres, and nylon stockings were among his favorites (although he also enjoyed donning his mother's robes when he was alone at home). Later, he substituted his wife's wardrobe, as he presently does. Daniel reports that his cross-dressing adventures have always had a high degree of erotic content, and that shame and humiliation are feelings that emerge *during* (rather than after) these episodes. His cross-dressing increases as opportunity allows and when other sexual activities are less frequent.

Unlike Daniel's sadomasochistic desires, Jeanie's did not develop until adulthood and marriage. She, in fact, sees such feelings as an outgrowth of her relationship with Daniel. She insists they were not a part of her childhood. In her words:

> Dan got me into S&M. Now I like it a lot. I never realized how much I could get into it but I sure do. Of course my feelings about Daniel helped. I love him. . . . At first I was confused and repulsed, but underneath I knew I had the potential for S&M in me.

Jeanie relates that she has recently come to prefer the masochistic role with Daniel, although that was not always the case. It was a "switch" in Daniel's preference that probably generated her own change. Although she is not fully aware of how the switch occurred with Daniel, she recognizes its importance for the present S&M arrangement between Daniel and herself.

In the absence of his wife, Daniel openly provides his account of how the change from masochist to sadist occurred in his mental life. Shortly after his marriage to Jeanie, Daniel found his masochistic desires increasingly difficult to suppress. Fearful of his new bride's negative reaction to the suggestion that they experiment with sadomasochism, Daniel began developing a relationship with a female co-worker who seemed promising:

> Brenda seemed like the type who would go for it. She dominated conversations and was hard and sometimes manish acting. She was cold but attractive, and hardly seemed naive about sex with men. I was sure she could get into dominating me, so I started an affair with her as soon as I got the chance.

Within the context of a series of clandestine encounters with his new mistress, Daniel gradually introduced sadomasochistic activities. He made attempts to persuade her to dominate him in several ways: with bondage, watersports, the administration of pain, and other S&M related practices. His mistress:

> just didn't have the heart for it. She surprised me, 'cause she wasn't the dominant type as I thought she would be. But I didn't give up, because something told me S&M was in her head somewhere.

As a final attempt, Daniel consciously decided to teach Brenda S&M dominance by demonstration. He himself practiced dominant sexual techniques on her:

> I started out easy, like with pinching her nipples. I spanked her a little, then I got tougher, screwing her as hard as I could. Then I got into humiliating her verbally, calling her a slut while I fucked her.

To Daniel's amazement, Brenda enjoyed these sessions more than she had any previous encounters. To his even greater amazement, Daniel discovered that he, too, was enjoying these S&M scenes. Along with his increasing pleasures as a master, their relationship grew stronger over a period of about two years. Daniel's affair was so intense that it began to interfere with his marriage. At this point, Daniel broke off the affair with Brenda. He describes this break:

> It was getting to be too much. I wasn't falling in love with her, but she was fulfilling my S&M needs so much. Actually, she was fulfilling my need to dominate, which I didn't even know I had until I started with her. I was growing dependent on her emotionally. It was starting to hurt my marriage and even my job. It was taking too much time too, so

I broke it off. By that time she was a real slave and I was a real master. Her submission fed my dominance and vice versa 'till it got to the point where little else occupied my head.

After his final meeting with Brenda, Daniel entered a period of erotic suppression. He held S&M desires and feelings at bay, spending more time and energy with his wife. Daniel found this arrangement satisfying for some time. Then, slowly at first, his S&M desires returned. This time, however, these desires were primarily dominant rather than submissive. His fantasies went in wild new directions, exploding into his mind's eye as never before. This switch in preference he attributes to his previous affair with Brenda:

By bringing out the bottom (masochist) in Brenda, I found out how great being a top (sadist) could be. She brought out my dominance at the same time. . . . Yeah, I guess I have a core-like slave in me, but being master turns me on too . . . especially with my wife now.

Presently, Daniel and Jeanie are discovering sadomasochism as never before. At the very beginning of their marriage, Jeanie unenthusiastically played the role of "top" in mild S&M scenes. Now, she finds far greater pleasure as a "bottom." Daniel also finds the new arrangement to his liking:

I'm getting her into being strongly dominated now and she responds beautifully. It's so beautiful that she amazes me with every encounter. It's terrific being married to someone who turns me on so intensely.

Daniel and Jeanie do not feel they have yet reached their limits in sadomasochism, but believe that the intensity of their feelings for each other will guide them safely to those limits. Sadomasochistic desires in the relationship between Daniel and Jeanie developed to their present state through a series of phases, beginning with marriage, the experimentation with Daniel as slave early in their marriage, Daniel's secret sexual episodes with Brenda, and finally with his dominance over his wife. As an indirect consequence of Daniel's lifelong sadomasochistic desires, his wife Jeanie eventually found and developed her own. These desires in adulthood thus emerged as a result of their emotional and erotic correspondence.

GLEN: PROFILE OF A TYPICAL GAY S&MER

Glen is not a particularly remarkable man in appearance, standing five-feet-seven-inches and weighing 150 pounds. He has rather handsome features, and is of masculine manner. Even his occupation as inventory clerk for a large northeastern manufacturer, and his midwestern, middle class background are not remarkable. What makes Glen different from others in his cohort is his homosexuality, and his interests in sadomasochism.

From the time Glen was five-years-old, he remembers having a sense of isolation from other members of his family. With his mother, he recalls, relations were distant. Glen was continually attempting to gain his mother's attention, but the struggle to make ends meet forced her to help her husband in his trade. Little time or energy was left to spend with Glen; but even the few moments shared with his mother were cool. Throughout his formative years, Glen recalls,

> my mother seldom had much time for me. She never looked me in the eyes or held me close like I wanted. She was always with my father who was a furniture refinisher. She usually did the shit-work he didn't want to do, like staining wood. She seemed to do the dirty work so willingly, but hardly spoke to me when I came around.

Interaction with his father was even less satisfactory for young Glen. Although he was normally considered a hard worker and good provider for his family, Glen's father experienced periods of drunkenness and violent behavior. These periods were marked by episodes of beatings and family life disruptions. According to Glen:

> All the time I was growing up, until I was twelve or thirteen, I was afraid of my father and his violent temper. Everyone in the family was afraid of him, but people outside the family figured he was a great guy. Outwardly he was fine, but when he was alone with his wife and us kids, he was hell. . . . We never knew when the violence would erupt, and there seemed to be no way to control it. We just waited in fear and anticipation of his arrival.

Glen recalls having several psychologically painful experiences with his father as well. These were generally characterized by hostility and an attempt to humiliate Glen. His father was especially cruel toward Glen's effeminacy. From a very early age, Glen was the object of such derogatory name-calling as "Daddy's sissy" and "the family faggot." One particularly memorable occasion occurred when Glen accompanied his father to a major league baseball game.

> I remember when I was ten, my father took me to a baseball game, something I always hated. I was bored to death, not caring about what I was watching. I tried not to show it by talking about the game like I was interested. I really liked it that he was taking me somewhere, and I didn't

want him to stop doing that. Without thinking about his reaction, I blurted out something about how awful I thought it was that the players were trampling the beautiful grass in the outfield. I asked my father why they had to play on the grass; and with a look of disgust, he asked me in a low voice if I knew what a faggot was. I said no, knowing that whatever it was, it was bad, and I must be one of them. I felt very odd and very much alone.

A profound feeling of being different stayed with Glen throughout his early years. This feeling was reinforced by two brothers who, Glen admits, usually wanted little to do with him, and by his sister, who avoided him entirely. Peers, too, played with him only long enough to mock him and oust him from his childhood activities. But it was not until later, when Glen was fifteen or so, that he came to realize the root cause of his feelings and manners. It was at that age that Glen found himself intensely attracted to a male classmate.

Glen's realization that he was homosexual led him to isolate himself from the outside world even more. While finishing high school, he concentrated on study and on his part-time job. Then, on the evening of his graduation from high school, Glen left his home and family behind. He took up residence in a western state, and continued to battle his homosexuality for several years.

In an attempt to defeat his homosexuality, Glen married at the age of twenty-three. But during three years of marriage, his attraction toward other males only intensified. At the same time that his wife began appealing to him for cooperation in starting a family, Glen finally realized that his homosexual feelings would not cease so easily. His divorce followed shortly after this realization. He then "came out" as openly gay to his family, admitting his homosexuality.

Glen was now twenty-five. Thus far sadomasochism had not been a part of Glen's homosexual feelings in any identifiable way. Other than fleeting adolescent erotic fantasies of bondage and constraint during sexual intercourse with another man, Glen had never thought about sadism and masochism.

S&M slowly entered Glen's sexual life. His first years of gay life were marked by rather conventional sexual activities. The newness and excitement of cruising and promiscuity precluded anything so sophisticated as sadomasochism. But the newness did not last.

S&M was always available to Glen during his initial experiences in the gay world. There were plenty of friends and acquaintances who were involved in S&M to some degree, and he knew where to find the local leather set. Glen first began patronizing leather bars in order to find masculine partners for sex. Many of the gay men he found in other bars were simply not masculine enough for him. Then, Glen explains,

I suddenly got out of gay life. Somehow it suddenly seemed cold and
cruel, superficial and dishonest. I was depressed and wanted nothing to
do with sex for a while. This lasted for a year or so. I guess I just got
burned out. . . . It wasn't turning me on anymore. . . . Something was
lacking.

Glen later began searching for that "something" among the S&M enthusiasts who frequented leather bars. As his curiosity about S&M developed,
Glen began asking himself questions such as which role he would be happiest
with, who would train him in S&M practices, and what his reactions would
be. His curiosity soon led to a series of initial encounters with a new friend
named Bill who:

taught me to be a slave and I loved it. It seemed so right for me that I
felt I had come home for the first time in my life. Serving him gave me
the warmest feelings I had ever had with anyone. It was great.

Since his first encounters with Bill and others, Glen has most often preferred the passive (insertee or "bottom") role. This preference has taken
many forms during sadomasochistic scenarios, including slave and master,
prisoner and warden (with a variation involving punk and wolf),[3] and even
innocent hitch-hiker and dirty old man.

As his experiences with sadomasochistic sex have accumulated, the goals
and meanings of such encounters have changed. Initially they were opportunities for sexual self-discovery. They served to "break the ice" and to
eliminate any residual guilt concerning his atypical sexual leanings. They
helped to shape his sexuality as well, both defining and discovering what he
found to be pleasurable. On this matter, Glen noted that "it is impossible to
say whether these scenes were erotic because they somehow expressed feelings I already had, or whether they actually created the feelings in the first
place."

Gradually, however, Glen came to find fulfillment in those encounters
which helped him discover the sexuality of his partners. It was this newer
practice of satisfying the needs of others that perhaps accounts for Glen's
emerging need to have a permanent S&M relationship. Glen describes this
need as he first felt it:

I found myself wanting someone to call my own after a few years of
this . . . in S&M. I wanted someone special. I guess I wanted to be a
slave to someone forever. I knew it was supposed to be hard for two
men to have a lasting relationship, but I wanted to try.

After several attempts to form a lasting relationship, Glen met his
present lover, Jim. Jim is extremely dominant, Glen explains, but loving

and, above all, caring. Glen has now spent the last four years as a slave to Jim, a period he describes as very satisfying:

> The last four years with Jim have been great. I've never felt so close to anyone in my life. We are able to communicate about everything, and his dominance over me has not become a way for him to take advantage, as it did with others. There are almost no jealousy trips and I feel 100 percent his. We are super in love.

The master and slave roles are generally confined to the bedroom. There is virtually no spillover into other areas of their relationship. Domestic decisions, chores, and responsibilities are shared equally. S&M roles, however, are almost never exchanged between Glen and Jim. Jim is always master. To have it otherwise, Glen explains, would disrupt the "fragile balance." That is, switching S&M roles would tend to destroy the images each has of the other, and thereby diffuse the auras of dominance and submission. For most S&M relationships, this diffusion is popularly thought to send shock waves throughout the delicate web of master-slave interactions. Both sexual and nonsexual arrangements would become problematic; they would again be strangers to each other's ways, yet they would have the added burden of a number of previously established expectations about each other's behavior. Like most other S&M couples, Glen and Jim have found it desirable to maintain their respective sex roles, while dispensing with them in other areas of their domestic life.

ROBBIE: A MASOCHISTIC BISEXUAL

Robbie is twenty-three years old. He is the second of six children. When he was seven or eight years old, his father left home. Robbie has not seen him since then. He was raised by his mother, with whom he feels especially close. He also reports feeling very close to his brothers and sisters.

Robbie remembers having been very unhappy during late grammar school. He was harassed by the other children at his parochial school; they labeled him a "faggot." At the time, he did not know what the word meant. In retrospect, Robbie thinks he might have been effeminate at that age, but he does not remember having noticed any feminine traits in himself. This was a very painful time. "When I was very young," he says, "I put myself in a shell. I had the feeling of being an outcast for a very long time." By his teens this seems to have changed, and Robbie says that he was happy as a teenager and fairly popular in high school. He attributes this later acceptance by his peers to their maturity and the development of more liberal attitudes.

Robbie's first sexual experience, at the age of sixteen, was with a man in his late twenties who had offered him a ride home from a concert. Robbie says that he enjoyed this encounter, but subsequent same-sex experiences were very infrequent during high school years.

At the age of seventeen, Robbie had his first sexual experience with a woman, who was a few years older than him. After this initial exposure to heterosexual relations, he began having sex on a regular basis with other women.

Robbie defines himself as bisexual, since he enjoys having sex with both men and women. Lately, though, he has been more sexually active with male partners. Despite having had some same-sex experiences in his late teens, Robbie claims that he has not been very attracted to men until relatively recently:

> I knew I'd go to bed with both sexes. One interesting thing is that I really did not look at men lustfully. Gay porno didn't turn me on. Straight porno did and still does . . . and then I look at gay porno and only if its well done in some ways aesthetically or maybe being kinky too, I may get turned on.

Robbie is a masochist. Ever since early childhood, he has had masochistic fantasies. Some of his thoughts are rather unusual. For example, in addition to having had both male and female oriented S&M fantasies with himself as the passive partner, Robbie has conceived scenarios within which he is manipulated by machines, masturbated by them, and subjected to their wishes.

When he was nineteen, Robbie left home to attend college in another state. It was then that he had his first sadomasochistic experience. His partner was an older man who was active in the city's gay community. This experience was exciting and pleasurable, Robbie says. It involved only "light" S&M: exhibitionism, mild slapping, and slight humiliation. Robbie reports that he was so excited about this episode that he was laughing. He says that his partner was "amazed" by Robbie's reaction, since the man knew that Robbie was a novice in S&M. This is a common response on the part of "masters." They are continually astonished by how masochistic their slaves are, how much punishment they can take, and how deeply they are involved in the scenario. The fact that the masochist gets pleasure from the same act as he does is perpetually astounding to the sadist.

Despite having had masochistic fantasies involving women, Robbie has never had an opportunity to act on them. He did, however, become friends with a sadistic woman:

> I met one S&M, sadistic-type woman in a bar in another city, but I never got into any S&M scenes with her because she said she could never

do it to somebody she was friends with. . . . I got along fairly well with her. It was very nice, actually. She introduced me to some interesting people. Eventually, I got involved with other things and stopped seeing her.

Robbie's experience illustrates the findings of Andreas Spengler, who found that the opportunity for heterosexual men to make S&M contacts was severely limited. Bisexuals, on the other hand, had a much better chance for realizing their desires, because they were willing to include other men as potential sex partners.

Robbie has a male friend with whom he regularly engages in sadomasochism. His friend, Robbie says, is a very good person and very affectionate. Although the other man can take both passive and aggressive parts, he is most often the master, since Robbie prefers to play slave.

Robbie enjoys being tied up (bondage) and whipped. The following portion of an interview with him nicely illustrates both his personal feelings about S&M and how the scene itself is a collaborative event, with the masochist having much of the control:

Interviewer: Do you go in for bondage?
Robbie: Um hum. Yes, I enjoy it very much.
I: Ropes, chains, or what?
R: Ropes, yeah. Could be anything.
I: Does he bind both your hands and feet?
R: That's the way its done.
I: Do you get hung at all?
R: I think I got hung once or twice.
I: Do you use any kind of paraphernalia?
R: He has leather thongs that he uses for whips, and also this dog leash that makes a pretty good whip.
I: Do you mind getting whipped? Do you like it?
R: I like it. I find that pretty stimulating.
I: What kinds of things do you anticipate doing or working up to doing?
R: I like getting bound and whipped, because that's what most of my fantasies are.
I: Do you set a limit on that, like how hard he can whip you or where?
R: Not consciously. He wanted to put a specific number on it and I said, "No, go ahead and do what you want."
I: He enjoys that too?
R: I think he does.
I: Do you ever whip him?
R: Uh huh. Yeah. He likes to change roles.

I: How do you feel about that?
R: Fairly neutral about that. It doesn't do a lot for me.

Robbie is also a transvestite, but he does not dress up as a woman during
S&M scenes. For those times, he wears a pair of bathing trunks that he has
shortened. He first began cross-dressing when he was nineteen or twenty.
He says that the desire to dress as a woman came upon him suddenly:

> One thing that did come suddenly was me becoming a transvestite. . . .
> This is something that's very clear in my mind. I started having dreams
> about transvestites for two nights in a row . . . and that gave me the
> idea I might enjoy it, so I tried it and I did.

Robbie was living back at home when he began to cross-dress. He found
some old clothes in the attic. At first, he put them on surreptitiously. Later,
he began to be more open about his interest. He became involved in a gay
organization and attended their dances and events dressed sometimes as a
woman and at other times in "gender fuck" (i.e., dressing so as to strike a
discordant note when viewed by "straight" people). He reports, for example, wearing a yellow chiffon dress and sporting a goatee at the same time.
Robbie does not define himself as a "drag queen."[5] He says that he is a
heterosexual transvestite. He reports getting sexual pleasure from dressing
up in women's clothing.

VITO: AN IDENTITY IN TRANSITION

Vito is twenty-one years old and a sophomore in college. He has dark eyes
and dark hair and is conventionally masculine in mannerisms and appearance. What is not conventional about Vito is his masochistic desires. These
are further intertwined with both homosexual and heterosexual interests.
During high school especially, Vito experienced a great deal of confusion
and psychological pain over his sexual feelings:

> I was kind of mixed up for a while. Kind of like really mixed up.
> Because I didn't know whether I wanted to get into a relationship with a
> guy or a girl and I was really hung up on my masochism. . . . I really
> didn't know where I was at sexually.

In an attempt to figure things out, Vito read "psychology" books mostly
and ordered books about homosexuality and masochism:

> I started reading a lot of books in late high school . . . just to discover

things. Like, I ordered these books through the mail. All my books were basically on homosexuals or masochists, those kind of things. Even then, I guess, I was worried about it.

Vito comes from a lower middle-class Italian family. He was born in a large eastern metropolis and moved to the suburbs when he was eight years old. He has one sister, three years younger than him. He characterizes his mother as being "overprotective." Vito indicates some fear of his father and sees himself as not measuring up to some masculine ideal that the latter represented. This deep-felt sense of inferiority affected his relationship with girls during high school. Although he did date, Vito felt uncomfortable around them:

> I was always kind of uptight about dates in high school. . . . I probably just felt nervous because, I guess, coming from my background, which is Italian culture—and my father, when he was younger, was into boxing, and also my grandfather was a construction worker—I think I always felt not manly enough. I always thought that if these girls really knew me, they wouldn't like me. I'm attracted to some girls, but I would like them to be the aggressor rather than me.

By the time he was about eleven years old, Vito had realized that he was attracted to males as well as to females. He did not act on this homosexual attraction, however, until he was much older. Vito recalls having had a crush on a best friend during high school, but he could never tell the other boy.

Vito had his first "petting" experience with a girl when he was thirteen. He met her at a party. She was the aggressor and allowed Vito to fondle her breasts. He felt very guilty about it afterward. Vito had a few other experiences with girls over the next few years, but they were limited to kissing and touching. He had not experienced sexual intercourse. At the age of eighteen, Vito decided to go to a prostitute:

> This was a different situation because, since I had gone out with a few girls and got really uptight with kissing and everything else, I figured that I should go to a prostitute and try something. . . . [It] was really a bad thing, because I didn't get off on it at all. And I think that after it, that's when I started saying, "you're definitely homosexual."

Vito began going to prostitutes to satisfy his masochistic desires. These scenes involved being verbally and physically humiliated and then masturbating. He did not have intercourse with these prostitutes. Vito says that he enjoyed these acts, but he did feel some guilt about them. It was also at about this time that Vito had his first homosexual experience. He met a young black man, in his mid-teens, with whom he established a sexual relationship. Unlike his previous relations with women, these homosexual experiences proved to be satisfying. "It was funny, when I got into it first, I might have been a little bit hung up about it. But then, that didn't last long, and I found the guy kind of attractive. So, I got into it."

At the age of nineteen, Vito had his first homosexual, sadomasochistic sexual experience. He had met a man at a meeting of an organization whose members included gay and heterosexual sadomasochists. Vito went home with the man and served as his slave. This initial exposure to gay S&M, however, proved to be disasterous for Vito. "With the prostitute I kind of liked it," Vito says, "but with this guy I didn't get into it at all."

Vito characterizes himself as "basically homosexual," but he is also interested in heterosexual relationships. He says that he is "fairly certain" about this. He stops short of considering himself bisexual, however, since he notes a greater attraction to men. Yet, he still finds himself attracted to women:

> Its funny. Most of the time I fantasize about guys; but there are times when I just look at a girl and fantasize about her. . . . I would definitely like to get into it if I could find the right woman.

Despite these fantasies, Vito is very wary of developing a heterosexual relationship. Some of his uncertainty lies in his feeling that he is not masculine enough. He is not an aggressive person and feels that this makes him unmanly. Encounters with females make him uncomfortable, because he feels that they expect him to be the aggressor:

> As of now, I'm still confused. . . . I don't know if I should go to a (gay) center and meet some guys or just meet some girl on campus. I really don't know. In a way, I'd rather meet up with some guy, because you don't have to worry about taking the initiative all the time or taking them out and buying them things. I'll see what happens, I guess. . . . Last semester, I definitely was interested in having a relationship with a few girls, but it just didn't work out.

Vito probably also recognizes that he has a greater probability of realizing his masochistic desires with men than with women. He did, in fact, note that the reason he went to prostitutes was that he assumed that most girls would reject him if he told them about his masochism.

Vito may have a long way to go in self-acceptance. He notes that he lacks self-confidence and that he feels insecure. He feels that his strong points include sincerity and being unprejudiced. Vito also has a lot of thinking to do about his sexual orientation. He has sought professional help in dealing with his feelings, but he does not believe that the psychologists whom he saw aided him very much. Given his ambivalence about women, it is quite probable that Vito will eventually become a participant in the gay S&M world, and limit his sexual activities to other men.

CONCLUSIONS

While the individual careers we have discussed are different in many ways there are, nevertheless, some common themes running through them. These similarities are all related to S&M as a form of social interaction. For example, the importance of learning both attitudes and techniques through a socialization process is evident in all of these careers. This is true even if an individual has had S&M fantasies from childhood as Daniel, Robbie, and Vito all report. Daniel relates that he first taught both Brenda and Jeanie how to dominate him, and then later he taught them how to be dominated. What he does not say, but what is implicit in his story, is that they, too, participated actively in the various scenarios and their responses taught him what did and did not work. Glen, Robbie, and Vito were all taught by persons who had previously been involved in S&M.

In order for an S&M scene to be successful, from the viewpoint of both partners, it must be collaboratively worked out. This is especially true for ongoing relationships like those reported by Daniel, Glen, and Robbie. Unless there is satisfaction on the part of both master (or mistress) and slave, the relationship will terminate. Thus, there must be agreement on the scene and consent given by both parties. Adjustments must be made by participants so that they are both stimulated. Vito's unhappy experience with a man is a case in point. In that situation only his partner was satisfied. Consequently, Vito was no longer willing to participate in S&M with this man. Robbie is fortunate in having a partner who can play both master and slave, since Robbie prefers the passive role. Yet, he also recognizes his friend's need to be dominated occasionally and, therefore, he will sometimes play master, even though, as he says, "It doesn't do a lot for me." Jeanie played the dominant role for Daniel for much the same reason.

Another finding apparent in all of these careers is that the S&M scene is a dynamic one with a constant feedback of "energy" between slave and master. This is most explicit when Daniel says of Brenda that, "her submission fed my dominance and vice versa." (Pat Galifia notes the same sort of "energy flow" in her article in this section.)

Finally, the importance of mutual love and affection for S&M couples is brought out by Daniel, Glen, and Robbie. They point out what sexologist Havelock Ellis noted long ago: that much sadomasochistic behavior is motivated by love.

REFERENCES

Califia, Pat, "A Secret Side of Lesbian Sexuality," *Advocate,* December 27, 1979: 19-23.

Ellis, Havelock, *Studies in the Psychology of Sex* (Vol. 1, Part 3), New York: Random House, 1942.

Goffman, Erving, *Stigma: Notes on the Management of Spoiled Identity,* Englewood Cliffs (N.J.): Prentice-Hall, 1963.

Spengler, Andreas, "Manifest Sadomasochism of Males: Results of an Empirical Study," *Archives of Sexual Behavior* 6: 441-456, 1977.

NOTE

1. "Fist-fucking" involves a technique whereby a hand penetrates the anal opening until the entire forearm is inserted into the anal cavity. This is done slowly and gently by inserting one finger at a time and carefully expanding the rectum.

2. We use the term "career" here in the way in which it has been defined by sociologist Erving Goffman: "Persons who have a particular stigma tend to have similar learning experiences regarding their plight, and similar changes in conception of self—a similar 'moral career' that is both cause and effect of commitment to a similar sequence of personal adjustments (*Stigma,* p. 32)."

3. "Punk" and "Wolf" are prison slang. A wolf is an aggressive, predatory man who takes the insertor role in anal sex, often as a rapist. He has a heterosexual self-identity. A "punk" is a weak, defensive victim, often small and young, who takes the passive sexual role. He is often heterosexual in orientation.

4. A "drag queen" is a homosexual man who dresses in women's clothing. His wardrobe and mannerisms are often exaggerated. Drag does not usually have a sexual meaning. It is often done for fun and humor.

Pat Califia

A Secret Side of Lesbian Sexuality

The sexual closet is bigger than you think. By all rights, we shouldn't be here, but we are. It's obvious that conservative forces like organized religion, the police, and other agents of the tyrannical majority don't want sadomasochism to flourish anywhere, and sexually active women have always been a threat the system won't tolerate. But conservative gay liberationists and orthodox feminists are also embarrassed by kinky sexual subcultures (even if that's where they do their tricking). "We are just like heterosexuals (or men)," is their plea for integration, their way of whining for some of America's carbon monoxide pie. Drag queens, leathermen, rubber freaks, boy-lovers, girl-lovers, dyke sadomasochists, prostitutes, transsexuals — we make that plea sound like such a feeble lie. We are not like everyone else. And our difference is not created solely by oppression. It is a preference, a sexual preference.

Lesbian S&M isn't terribly well-organized (yet). But in San Francisco, women can find partners and friends who will aid and abet them in pursuing the delights of dominance and submission. We don't have bars. We don't even have newspapers or magazines with sex ads. I sometimes think the gay subculture must have looked like this, when urbanization first started. Since our community consists of word-of-mouth and social networks, we have to work very hard to keep it going. It's a survival issue. If the arch-conformists with their cardboard cunts and angora wienies had their way, we wouldn't exist at all. As we become more visible, we encounter more hostility, more violence. This article is my way of refusing the narcotic of self-hatred. We must break out of the silence that persecution imposes on its victims.

I am a sadist. The polite term is "top," but I don't like to use it. It dilutes my image and my message. If someone wants to know about my sexuality, they can deal with me on my own terms. I don't particularly care to make it easy. S&M is scary. That's at least half its significance. We select the most frightening, disgusting, or unacceptable activities and transmute them into pleasure. We make use of all the forbidden symbols and all the disowned emotions. S&M is a deliberate, premeditated, erotic blasphemy. It is a form of sexual extremism and sexual dissent.

I identify more strongly as a sadomasochist than as a lesbian. I hang out in the gay community because that's where the sexual fringe starts to unravel. Most of my partners are women, but gender is not my boundary. I am limited by my own imagination, cruelty and compassion, and by the greed and stamina of my partner's body. If I had a choice between being shipwrecked on a desert island with a vanilla lesbian and a hot male masochist, I'd pick the boy. This is the kind of sex I like—sex that tests physical limits within a context of polarized roles. It is the only kind of sex I am interested in having.

I am not typical of S&M lesbians, nor do I represent them. In fact, because I define myself as a sadist, I am atypical. Most S&M people *prefer* the submissive "bottom" or masochistic role. The bulk of the porn (erotic, psychoanalytic, and political) that gets written about S&M focuses on the masochist. People who do public speaking about S&M have told me they get a more sympathetic hearing if they identify as bottoms. This makes sense, in a twisted kind of way. The uninitiated associate masochism with incompetence, lack of assertiveness, and self-destruction. But sadism is associated with chainsaw murders. A fluffy-sweater type listening to a masochist may feel sorry for her, but she's terrified of me. I'm the one who is ostensibly responsible for manipulating or coercing the M into degradation—all 130 pounds 5' 2" of me. Therefore, my word is suspect. It is nevertheless true that my services are in demand, that I respect my partners' limits and that both (or more) of us obtain great pleasure from a scene. I started exploring S&M as a bottom, and I still put my legs in the air now and then. I have never asked a submissive to do something I haven't or couldn't do.

In addition to being a sadist, I have a leather fetish. If I remember my Krafft-Ebing, that's another thing women aren't supposed to do. Oh, well. Despite the experts, seeing, smelling, or handling leather makes me cream. Every morning before I go out the door, I make a ritual out of putting on my leather jacket. The weight of it, settling on my shoulders, is reassuring. Once I zip it, turn the collar up and cram my hands into the pockets, the jacket is my armor. It also puts me in danger when I wear it on the street by alerting the curious and the angry to my presence.

I get all kinds of different reactions. Voyeurs drool. Queer-baiting kids shout or throw bottles from their cars. Well-dressed hets,* secure in their privilege, give me the condescending smile of the genital dilettante. Some gay men are amused when they see me coming. They take me for a fag hag,* a mascot dressed up to avoid embarrassing my macho friends. Others are resentful. Leather is their province, and a cunt is not entitled to wear the insignia of a sadomasochist. They avoid my shadow. I might be menstruating and make their spears go dull. When I visit a dyke bar, the patrons take me for a member of that nearly-extinct species, the butch. Femmes under this misapprehension position themselves within my reach, signaling their availability, not bothering to actively pursue me. They seem to expect me to do everything a man would do, except knock them up. Given the fact that I prefer someone to come crawling and begging for my attention, and to work pretty damned hard before they get it, this strikes me as being very funny. In women's groups, the political clones, the Dworkinites,† see my studded belt and withdraw. I am obviously a sex pervert, and good, real true lesbians are not sex perverts. They are high priestesses of feminism, conjuring up the "wimmin's" revolution. As I understand it, after the wimmin's revolution, sex will consist of wimmin holding hands, taking their shirts off and dancing in a circle. Then we will all fall asleep at exactly the same moment. If we didn't all fall asleep, something else might happen—something male-identified, objectifying, pornographic, noisy, and undignified. Something like an orgasm.

This is why they say leather is expensive. When I wear it, disdain, amusement, and the threat of violence follow me from my door to my destination and home again. Is it worth it? Can the sex be that good? When am I going to get to the point and tell you what we do?

I can smell your titillation. Well—since you want it so bad, I'll let you have a taste of it.

If I'm interested in someone, I call them up and ask them if they'd like to go out for dinner. I have never picked up a stranger in a bar. My partners are friends, women who strike up acquaintances with me because they've heard me talk about S&M, women I know from Samois.‡ (I also have a lover who is my slave. We enjoy conducting joint seductions or creating bizarre sexual adventures to tell each other about later.) If she agrees, I will tell her where and when to meet me. Over dinner, I begin to play doctor—Dr. Kinsey. I like to know when she started being sexual with other people, if and when she started masturbating, if and how she likes to have an

---

*"het," slang for heterosexual—*Eds.*

*"fag hag," a heterosexual woman who associates extensively with male homosexuals—*Eds.*
†Dworkinites are followers of Andrea Dworkin, an activist in Women Against Pornography. She has often been criticized for what have been perceived as anti-male and anti-sexual attitudes—*Eds.*
‡Samois is a support group for lesbians interested in S&M, located in the San Francisco Bay area—*Eds.*

orgasm, when she came out as a lesbian (if she has), and I give her similar information about me. Then I like to ask about her S&M fantasies and how much experience she has with acting them out. I also try to find out if she has any health problems (asthma, diabetes, etc.) that should limit play.

This conversation need not be clinical. It is not an interview—it is an interrogation. I am taking for granted my right to possess intimate information about my quarry. Giving me that information is the beginning of her submission. The sensations this creates are subtle, but we both begin to get turned on.

I will probably encourage her to get a little high. I don't like playing with women who are too stoned to feel what I am doing, nor do I want someone shedding inhibitions because of a chemical they've ingested. I prefer to deny a bottom any inhibitions and to take them away. However, I do like her to feel relaxed and somewhat vulnerable and suggestible.

If there's time, we may go to a bar. Socializing in gay men's leather bars is problematic for a lesbian. I prefer bars where I know some of the bartenders and patrons. I have rarely been refused admittance, but I have been made uncomfortable by men who felt I was an intruder. If there were women's bars that didn't make me feel even more unwelcome, I'd go there. Since I am a sadomasochist, I feel entitled to the space I take up in a men's bar. I sometimes wonder how many of the men exhibiting their leather in the light from the pinball machines go home and really work it out, and how many of them settle for fucking and sucking.

A leather bar provides a safe place to start establishing roles. I like to order my submissive to bring me a drink. She doesn't get a beer of her own. When she wants a drink, she asks me for one, and I pour it into her mouth while she kneels at my feet. I begin to handle her, appraising her flesh, correcting her posture, and fondling or exposing her so that she feels embarrassed and draws closer to me. I like to hear someone ask for mercy or protection. If she isn't already wearing a collar, I put one on her, and drag her over to a mirror—behind the bar, in the bathroom, on a wall—and make her look at it. I watch the response very carefully. I don't like women who collapse into passivity, whose bodies go limp and faces go blank. I want to see the confusion, the anger, the turn-on, the helplessness.

As soon as I am sure she is turned on (something that can be ascertained with the index finger if I can get her zipper down), I hustle her out of there. I especially like to put someone in handcuffs and lead them out on a leash.

This is one of the gifts I offer a submissive: the illusion of having no choice, the thrill of being taken.

The collar will keep her aroused until we reach my flat. I prefer to play in my space since it's set up for bondage and whipping. I will order her to stay two steps behind me, to reassure her that we really are going to do a scene. As soon as the door is locked behind us, I order her to strip. In my room, there is no such thing as casual nudity. When I take away someone's clothing, I am temporarily denying their humanity, with all its privileges and responsibilities.

Nudity can be taken a step further. The bottom can be shaved. A razor, passing over the skin, removes the pelt that warms and conceals. My lover/slave has her cunt shaved. It reminds her that I own her genitals, and reinforces her role as my child and property.

Shedding her clothes while I remain fully dressed is enough to shame and excite most bottoms. Once she is naked, I put her on the floor, and there she stays until I move her or raise her up. I stand over her, trail a riding crop down her spine, and tell her that she belongs underneath me. I talk about how good she's going to make my cunt feel and how strict I am going to be with her. I may allow her to embrace my boots. After delineating her responsibilities and cussing her out a little for being easy, I haul her up, slap her face, hold her head against my hip while I unzip, and let her feast on my clit.

I wonder if any man could understand how this act, receiving sexual service, feels to me. I was taught to dread sex, to fight it off, to provide it under duress or in exchange for romance and security. I was trained to take responsibility for other people's gratification and pretend pleasure when others pretend to have my pleasure in mind. It is shocking and profoundly satisfying to commit this piece of rebellion, to take pleasure exactly as I want it, to exact it like tribute. I need not pretend I enjoy a bottom's ministration if they are unskilled, nor do I need to be grateful.

I like to come before I do a scene because it takes the edge off my hunger. For the same reason, I don't like to play when I am stoned or drunk. I want to be in control. I need all my wits about me to outguess the bottom's needs and fears, take her out of herself, and bring her back. During the session, she will receive much more direct physical stimulation than I will. So I take what I need. From her mouth, she feeds me the energy I need to dominate and abuse her.

While I am getting off, I usually begin to fantasize about the woman on her knees. I visualize her in a certain position or a certain role. This fantasy is the seed that the whole scene sprouts from. When she's finished pleasing me, I order her to crawl onto my bed, which is on the floor, and I tie her up.

Bottoms tend to be anxious. Because there is a shortage of tops, they get used to playing all kinds of little psychological numbers on themselves to feel miserable and titillated. They also like to feel greedy and guilty, and get anxious about that. The bondage is reassurance. She can measure the intensity of my passion by the tightness of my knots. It also puts an end to bullshit speculation about whether I am doing this just because she likes it so much. I make sure there's no way she can get loose on her own. Restraint becomes security. She knows I want her. She knows I am in charge.

Being tied up is arousing, and I intensify this arousal by teasing her, playing with her breasts and clit, calling her nasty names. When she starts to squirm, I begin to rough her up a little, taking her to the edge of pain, the edge that melts and turns over into pleasure. I move from pinching her nipples to a pair of clamps that makes then ache and burn. I may put clips all over her breasts or on the labia. I will check her cunt to make sure it's still wet, and tell her how turned on she is, if she doesn't already know.

At some point, I will always use a whip. Some bottoms like to be whipped until they are bruised. Others find just the visual image exciting and may want to hear the sound of it whistling in the air or feel the handle moving in and out of them. A whip is a great way to get someone to be here now. They can't look away from it, and they can't think about anything else.

If the pain goes beyond a mild discomfort, the bottom will probably get scared. She will start to wonder, "Why am I doing this? Am I going to be able to take this?" There are many ways to get someone past this point. One is to ask her to take it for me because I need to watch her suffer. One is to administer a fixed number of blows as a punishment for some sexual offense. Another is to convince a bottom that they deserve the pain, and must endure it because they are "only" a slave. Pacing is essential. The sensations need to increase gradually. The particular implement involved may also be important. Some women who cannot tolerate whipping have a very high tolerance for other things—nipple play, hot wax, enemas, or verbal humiliation.

When I am playing bottom, I don't want pain or bondage for their own sake. I want to please. The top is my mistress. She has condescended to train me, and it is very important to me to deserve her attention. The basic dynamic of S&M is the power dichotomy, not pain. Handcuffs, dog collars, whips, kneeling, being bound, tit clamps, hot wax, enemas, penetration, and giving sexual service are all metaphors for the power imbalance. However, I must admit that I get bored pretty fast with a bottom who is not willing to take any pain.

The will to please is a bottom's source of pleasure, but it is also a source of danger. If the top's intentions are dishonorable (i.e., emotional sabotage) or her skill is faulty, the bottom is not safe when she yields. The primary point of competition among tops is to be emotionally and physically safe to play with, to be worthy of the gift of submission. Someone who makes mistakes gets a bad reputation very fast, and only inexperienced or foolish bottoms will go under for them.

Why would anyone want to be dominated, given the risks? Because it is a healing process. As a top, I find the old wounds and unappeased hunger I nourish, I cleanse and close the wounds. I devise and mete out appropriate punishments for old, irrational sins. I trip the bottom up, I see her as she is, and I forgive her and turn her on and make her come, despite her unworthiness or self-hatred or fear. We are all afraid of losing, of being captured and defeated. I take the sting out of that fear. A good scene doesn't end with orgasm—it ends with catharsis.

I would never go back to tweaking tits and munching cunt in the dark, not after this. Two lovers sweating against each other, each struggling for her own goal, eyes blind to each other—how appalling, how deadly. I want to see and share in every sensation and emotion my partner experiences, and I want all of it to come from me. I don't want to leave anything out. The affronted modesty and the hostility are as important as the affection and lust.

The bottom must be my superior. She is the victim I present for the night's inspection. I derive an awful knowledge from each gasp, the tossing head, the blanching of her knuckles. In order to force her to lose control, I must unravel her defenses, breach her walls, and alternate subtlety and persuasion with brutality and violence. Playing a bottom who did not demand my respect and admiration would be like eating rotten fruit.

S&M is high technology sex. It is so time consuming and absorbing that I have no desire to own anyone on a full-time basis. I am satisfied with their sexual submission. This is the difference between real slavery or exploitation and S&M. I am interested in something ephemeral, pleasure, not in economic control or forced reproduction.

This may be why S&M is so threatening to the established order, and why it is so heavily penalized and persecuted. S&M roles are not related to gender or sexual orientation or race or class. My own needs dictate which role I will adopt. Our political system cannot digest the concept of power unconnected to privilege. S&M recognizes the erotic underpinnings of our systems, and seeks to reclaim them. There's an enormous hard-on beneath the priest's robe, the cop's uniform, the president's business suit, the soldier's khakis. But that phallus is powerful only as long as it is concealed, elevated to the level of a symbol, never exposed or used in literal fucking. A cop with his hard on sticking out can be punished, rejected, blown, or you can sit on it, but he is no longer a demi-god. In an S&M context, the uniforms and roles and dialogue become a parody of authority, a challenge to it, a recognition of its secret sexual nature.

Governments are based on sexual control. Any group of people who gain access to authoritarian power become accessories to that ideology. They begin to perpetuate and enforce sexual control. Women and gays who are hostile to other sexual minorities are siding with fascism. They don't want the uniforms to degenerate into drag—they want uniforms of their own.

As I write this, there is a case in Canada that will determine whether or not S&M sex between consenting adults can be legal. This case began when a gay male bathhouse that caters to an S&M clientele was raided. After that raid, a man in Toronto was busted for "keeping a common bawdy house." The "bawdy house" was a room in his apartment he had fixed up for S&M sex. Yet another man was busted for false imprisonment and aggravated assault. These charges stemmed from an S&M three-way.*

---

*As of early 1983, a number of these cases were still slowly being processed through the courts. Jim Bartley, in an article entitled "Morality: Fishing for Victims," appearing in the January 1983 issue of *Body Politic* (Toronto's gay newspaper), notes that ninety percent of the cases have resulted in acquittal. —*Eds.*

In San Francisco, months before Moscone and Milk were assassinated and the cops smashed into the Elephant Walk, half the leather bars in the Folsom Street area lost their liquor licenses due to police harassment. The Gay Freedom Day Parade Committee tried to pass a resolution that would bar leather and S&M regalia from the parade.

I don't know how long it will take for other S&M people to get as angry as I am. I don't know how long we will continue to work in gay organizations that patronize us and threaten us with expulsion if we don't keep quiet about our sexuality. I don't know how long we will continue to let women's groups who believe that S&M and pornography are the same thing and cause violence against women to go unchallenged because they are ostensibly feminist. I don't know how long we will continue to run our sex ads in magazines that feature judgmental, slanderous articles about us. I don't know how long we will continue to be harassed and assaulted or murdered on the street, or how long we will tolerate the fear of losing our apartments or being fired from our jobs or arrested for making the wrong kind of noise during some heavy sex.

I do know that whenever we start to get angry, walk out, and work for our own cause, it will be long overdue.

Gerhard Falk and Thomas S. Weinberg

Sadomasochism and Popular Western Culture

Traditionally, sadomasochism (S&M) has been studied as an individual psychopathology (Krafft-Ebbing, 1932; Freud, 1938). Recently, however, members of the medical (Spengler, 1977), sociological (Weinberg, 1978; Weinberg and Falk, 1980), and journalistic (Coburn, 1977; Halpern, 1977; Smith and Cox, 1979a, 1979b) professions have begun to examine S&M as a social behavior. The work of these writers has focused upon sado-masochism as a unique subculture, examining how the people within it make contacts, how S&M organizations function, and so forth. The present paper takes an even broader view of sadomasochism, examining the ways in which this behavior has become more visible within the culture of the larger society. Sadomasochistic themes are found throughout Western culture; they are not unique to "deviant" subcultures, although these themes are most highly developed and elaborated within them. In this paper we will be focusing on sadomasochism as a (1) sexual, (2) consensual, and (3) recreational phenomenon. We are eliminating from our discussion examples that do not include these three elements.

HISTORICAL ASPECTS

The history of sadomasochism as an erotic, consensual, and recreational behavior can be traced back at least two hundred years to eighteenth-and nineteenth-century England. During that period of time, private clubs, whose members often enjoyed whipping and birching as a form of recreation,

---

*Specially written for the present volume.

abounded in London. The "Hell-Fire Club," composed of men and "The Order of St. Bridget," whose members were women, engaged extensively in whipping, giving rise to the works of Leopold von Sacher-Masoch and influencing the writing of the English historian Thomas Buckle on the same subject (Bullough, 1976, p. 479).

English schools were devoted to the use of "birch discipline" and the "learned Dr. Johnson was an ardent advocate of the birch" (White, 1950, p. 84). White writes in *The Age of Scandal* that the headmaster of Eaton, Dr. Keate, "flogged more than eighty boys in one day," and that Lawrence, the great Governor-General of India, was flogged every day (pp. 86-87). A Dr. Parr and others are reported to have flogged the bottoms of students for failure to answer questions in school (White, 1950, p. 84).

The philosopher Jean-Jacques Rousseau related in his *Confessions* that as a boy he was sent to a boarding school where the sister of the director spanked him. He enjoyed this so much that he deliberately provoked further spankings and, in his adult life, he consciously sought out women who would be willing to spank him (Rousseau, 1935, p. 19).

EIGHTEENTH-AND NINETEENTH-CENTURY S&M LITERATURE

A variety of sadomasochistic literature appeared and was circulated in the eighteenth and nineteenth centuries. In 1810, George Colman wrote a poem called the "Rodiad," in which he praises flogging as a kind of recreation or "sport." The final few verses of that poem read,

> Delightful sport! whose never failing charm
> Makes young blood tingle and keeps old blood warm—
> From you I have no fancy to repair
> To where *unbottomed* Cherubs haunt the air;
> Rather, methinks, I could with better grace
> Present myself at some inferior place—
> There offer, without salary to pursue,
> The business that on earth I best could do—
> Propose to scourge the diabolic flesh,
> Forever tortured and forever fresh;
> Cut up with red-hot wire adulterous Queens,
> Man-burning Bishops, Sodomizing Deans,
> Punish with endless pain a moment's crime,
> and whip the wicked out of space and time;
> Nor if the "Eternal Schoolmaster" is stern
> And dooms me to correction in my turn
> Shall I complain. When better hope is past
> Flog and be flogged is no bad fate at last.
> (Fraxi, 1962, p. 474)

In his *Bibliography of Prohibited Books,* Pisanus Fraxi (1962) lists numerous volumes that describe a variety of spanking, beating, and whipping scenes, all occurring in England during those two centuries. One publication, for instance, which was privately printed, describes the whipping of female culprits at Bridewell prison in the eighteenth century (Fraxi, 1962, p. 443); another, *The Memoirs of John Bell,* relates the experiences of a domestic servant who worked for a widow who enjoyed whipping children (p. 459); while the play "The Virtuoso," by Thomas Shadwell, depicts a protagonist who comes to a prostitute to be flogged (p. 450). In the third volume of Fraxi's book, there appear "Experimental Lecture by Col. Spanker" (p. 246), "Curiosities of Flagellation" (p. 251), and "The Quintessence of Birch Discipline" (p. 258). An excerpt in the memoirs of *Fanny Hill* (Cleland, 1965), originally published in the middle of the eighteenth century,* describes how a prostitute whips a "gentleman" and is, in turn, beaten by him (Cleland, 1965, pp. 172–181).

The best known works dealing with sadomasochistic themes in the last century were not, however, written in the English language. Most prominent among these novels were the Marquis de Sade's *Justine* (1976) and *Juliette* (1966)† and Leopold von Sacher-Masoch's (1978) *Venus in Furs.* It was, of course, from the names of these writers that Krafft-Ebing coined the terms "sadism" and "masochism."

SADOMASOCHISM AND MODERN POPULAR CULTURE

Eighteenth- and nineteenth-century sadomasochistic clubs and literature have their modern counterparts (Weinberg and Falk, 1980). Sadomasochistic themes are found not only in books, but in movies and music as well. Explicit S&M material in contemporary culture, however, seems to be more widely disseminated than it was in the last century. It is now more available to a general audience rather than being confined to an erotic elite. Judging by the rise of S&M "boutiques" and "adult toy" shops in the larger cities, such as the "Pleasure Chest" in New York City, and sadomasochistic depictions in popular fashion magazines, one journalist concluded that there is now an "S&M chic" (Coburn, 1977). Sadomasochism, however, is more than just "chic"; it is part of the recreational activities of many Americans. This can be seen through a brief survey of some of the more popular movies, literature, and music.

Fanny Hill was privately printed in 1749. However, there is some dispute as to the original publisher. There is some evidence that the manuscript was privately circulated prior to this date.
†*Juliette* was originally published in 1796. *Justine* was first published in 1791.

Movies with Sadomasochistic Themes

There are many explicitly erotic S&M scenes in movies shown in this country. Spanking scenes have been part of many films, even those made in the forties and fifties. In the majority of these movies, women are spanked by men. Among such films are *Kiss Me Kate, Eve: the Diary of a Young Girl,* and *Captain Lightfoot* (deCoulteray, 1965, p. 93). In some movies, however, women spank women (e.g., *Two Women,* and *Man and Child*) and in others such as *The Young Wolves* and *Eva,* women beat men. In the latter two movies, the aggressor woman is depicted as wearing high boots and carrying a riding crop (deCoulteray, 1965, p. 109), a common S&M motif. A more recent movie, *The Choirboys,* has a scene in which a professional dominatrix whips a man who is bound, gagged, and has his face covered with a leather mask. The same sort of sadomasochistic theme is played for laughs in another contemporary movie, *Wholly Moses,* in which knowledge of S&M is treated as a joke whose humor the film makers took for granted would be understood and appreciated by a mass audience. In this movie, the hero enters "New Sodom" and observes an S&M puppet show, complete with a cat-o-nine-tails wielding marionette "dominatrix" and her male "slave."

The sexual aspect of sadomasochism is more explicitly shown in scenes of women using dildoes to anally rape or copulate with men such as in *Myra Breckenridge* and *The Opening of Misty Beethoven,* a behavior and theme very prevalent in the American S&M subculture.[1] The frequency with which spanking and similar scenes appear in both American and foreign movies would seem to indicate that they are appreciated by American audiences.[2]

In addition to movies that include sadomasochistic scenes, there are those based upon S&M themes. *The Story of O,* Pauline Réage's (1966) novel inspired a movie that has been appearing in neighborhood theaters for the last few years. This film along with *Venus in Furs,* the Sacher-Masoch (1978) account of a masochistic man's obsession with a woman who treats him cruelly, and the now classic *The Night Porter* have been shown on the "adult" channels of pay television. Both *Venus in Furs* and *The Night Porter* explore the psychological as well as the physically erotic aspects of S&M.

Modern Sadomasochistic Literature and Music

In addition to movies, there are large numbers of books describing an endless variety of beatings, spankings, and whippings. The most graphic is Robert Briffault's (1935, pp. 301–303) description of the whipping of a noble Russian woman in *Europa.* Other examples are *Under the Hill* by

Aubrey Beardsley (1904)*, who describes the birching of a girl and a boy by two older women, and *Confessions and Experiences* by Edith Cadivec (1971), which describes the author's erotic feelings in connection with birching by another woman. In *New At It,* Blake Tremain (1973) describes the caning of a boy by a young woman, and in *The Image,* Jean deBerg (1966) relates the story of a young man who becomes increasingly more involved in the sadomasochistic relationship between two women.

Although songs about rejection by "cruel" lovers have been popular for decades, they were not really "sadomasochistic" in the sense that we have been using the term in this paper. More recently, however, S&M ideas have become more apparent, most notably in rock music. For example, part of the promotion for the Rolling Stones' album, *Black and Blue,* featured a billboard picturing a young woman, bruised and bound hand and foot. Indeed, some of the songs performed by this group, most notably "Under My Thumb," explicitly state S&M themes.[3] Other performers, such as singer Alice Cooper, have included sadomasochistic motifs in their stage shows. A number of "punk rock" bands of the 1980s appear in black leather, chains, and other S&M trappings, while some "New Wave" groups such as the Vibrators ("Whips and Furs" and "I Need a Slave") and Soft Cell ("Sex Dwarf") record songs that are overtly sadomasochistic.

Conclusions

Although sadomasochism is manifested in many areas of popular culture, rather than being limited to an erotic underground, the majority of people exposed to this material, probably take only a vicarious part in it. Others, undoubtedly, simply do not perceive any erotic content in it at all. Still other consumers of this material take an active role in pursuing S&M contacts. For these individuals, participation in sadomasochistic activities is very definitely a kind of sexual recreation. This can be seen from even a casual perusal of ads in sadomasochistic contact publications:

1. Why be lonely in New York? Have well-equipped flat and if you enjoy good music, wine, and an unusual evening with an imaginative mistress, send phone for fast reply.
2. Dominating female wants to meet couples and bi-gals who enjoy chained restraint, B&D, fun and games. Also enjoy French, Greek, and water sports. Have dominant or submissive male partners if desired.

---

*In an editors' note to an excerpt of *Under the Hill,* appearing in the appendix of their *S/M: The Last Taboo* (New York: Grove Press, 1974.), Gerald and Caroline Greene state that this work was incomplete at the time of Beardsley's death in 1898. The excerpt included by the Greenes was part of a posthumous collection published in 1904. —*Eds.*

3. Bi-gal with kinky husband seeks couples and gals. Both dig bizarre photography, restrictive costumes. We'll swing, watch you or watch us.

Recreation as an institution has become increasingly important in the modern Western societies of England, France, Germany, Canada, and the United States, as both affluence and leisure time increase. An interesting concomitant of the development of leisure time has been the redefinition of sexual behavior as "play." The broadening of acceptable modes of sexual expression has included erotic pain, so that sadomasochism is defined by many people as a form of sexual recreation.[4]

NOTES

1. See, for example, Halpern (1977). Volume 2, Number 12 of *Latent Image* has a letter from a male submissive reader who writes, in part, "some mistresses, bringing to the surface those latent resentments that most females suppress, find the urge to turn the tables more completely, visiting upon their helpless subject, bound in receptive position and perhaps well gagged and even blindfolded to taunt him with his forced docility, the privilege of penetration and possession at will. What men for centuries have considered their right, regardless of the desires and feelings of their wives and girlfriends, becomes sweet revenge when the dildo is on the other body." The same volume contains a photo of a "beautiful dominatrix" who is masked and in high heeled boots. In her left hand she is holding a cat-o-nine-tails, and around her hips she wears a dildo complete with testicles.
2. Even non-S&M oriented movies can, of course, be treated as if they were intentionally sadomasochistic. A writer in *Amazon* (no. 8, p. 67), an S&M contact magazine, for example, tells the publication's readers: "Here's a tip, as we say adieu: Valerie Perrine, in her (censored) costumes, is worth whatever the ticket price to SUPERMAN may be in the area you live in. We'd have paid the full price just to see her!"
3. For example, in this song the singer describes how a woman who had formerly "pushed him around" is now under his complete domination and control. He likens her to a "squirming dog," a common S&M motif; and he demonstrates his power over her by noting that he determines her behavior: when she speaks, where she casts her eyes, and even the clothing she wears.
4. In a recent unpublished manuscript, Martha S. Magill (1982) suggests that sadomasochism may be profitably explained by using anthropological play theory.

REFERENCES

Berg, Jean de. *The Image.* New York: Grove Press, 1966.

Briffault, R. *Europa: The Days of Ignorance.* New York: Charles Scribner's Sons, 1935.

Bullough, Vern L. *Sexual Variance in Society and History.* New York: John Wiley & Sons, 1976.

Cadivec, Edith. *Confessions and Experiences.* New York: Grove Press, 1971.

Cleland, John. *Fanny Hill, The Memoirs of a Woman of Pleasure.* New York: New American Library, 1965.

Coburn, Judith. "S&M," *New Times* 8 (February 4): 43, 45-50, 1977.

deCoulteray, G. *Sadism in the Movies.* New York: The Medical Press, 1965.

Fraxi, Pisanus. *Bibliography of Prohibited Books.* New York: Jack Brussel Publishers, 1960.

Freud, Sigmund. *The Basic Writings of Sigmund Freud.* (A. A. Brill, trans. and ed.). New York: The Modern Library, 1938.

Halpern, Bruce. "Spanks for the Memory," *Screw* 420 (March 21): 4-7, 1977.

Krafft-Ebing, R. von. *Psychopathia Sexualis.* New York: Physicians' and Surgeons' Book Co., 1932.

Magill, M. S. "Ritual and Symbolism of Dominance and Submission: The Case of Heterosexual Sadomasochism," unpublished manuscript, Department of Anthropology, State University of New York at Buffalo, 1982.

Réage, Pauline. *Story of O.* New York: Grove Press, 1966.

Rousseau, J. J. *The Confessions of Jean-Jacques Rousseau.* (W. Conyngham Mallory, trans.). New York: Tudor Publishing Co., 1935.

Sacher-Masoch, Leopold von. *Venus in Furs.* New York: Privately printed for subscribers only (illustrated by Charles Raymond), 1928.

Sade, Donatien Alphonse, Francois de. *Juliette.* New York: Grove Press, 1976.

————. *Justine, Philosophy in the Bedroom, Eugenie de Franval, and Other Writings.* New York: Grove Press, 1966.

Smith, Howard and Cathy Cox. "Scenes: S&M in the Open," *Village Voice* 24 (January 15): 24, 1979a.

————. "Scenes: Dialogue with a Dominatrix," *Village Voice* 24 (January 29): 19-20, 1979b.

Spengler, Andreas. "Manifest Sadomasochism of Males: Results of an Empirical Study" *Archives of Sexual Behavior* 6: 441-456, 1977.

Tremaine, Blake. *New At It.* New York: Grove Press, 1973.

Weinberg, T. S. "Sadism and Masochism: Sociological Perspectives." *Bulletin of the American Academy of Psychiatry and the Law* 6: 284-299, 1978.

Weinberg, T. S. and Gerhard Falk, "The Social Organization of Sadism and
    Masochism," *Deviant Behavior* 1 (July/Sept.): 379–393, 1980.
White T. H. *The Age of Scandal.* London: Jonathan Cape & Co., 1950.

STRUCTURES
THE SOCIAL ORGANIZATION
OF S&M

Introduction

"The Social Organization of Sadism and Masochism" by Weinberg and Falk begins our third section, which is concerned with *structures*. It expands our exploration of sadomasochism to a broader level of examination by discussing important features of its social organization. Focusing upon heterosexual S&M, this essay illuminates mechanisms for finding contacts, avenues for sex education and informed communication available to primarily nonhomosexual S&Mers, and the functions of organizational sadomasochism.

While some ideas on identity and S&M scenes are included in G. W. Levi Kamel's discussion of "Leathersex," this contribution focuses primarily on sadomasochism as an organized subculture. Rather than view S&M stereotypically as randomly violent behavior, Kamel shows that it is a highly prescribed, normatively controlled, and rationally accomplished sociosexual activity. It is, in a word, socially *meaningful* behavior among its participants. Some of the tenets of existential sociology are implicit throughout the essay.

"The Social Organization of Sexual Risk" by John Alan Lee also focuses upon the social organization of gay S&M. While similar in many ways to Kamel's work — primarily because both writers are concentrating on a very specifically bounded and well-developed culture — Lee examines several exciting new issues that are also of scientific importance. For example, he discusses the political significance of S&M for other social behavior in terms of power dimensions.

Another feature of Lee's essay is that it is theoretically nurtured throughout, again using the dramaturgical mode of analysis. He thus brings further along in its development as a useful analytical tool the suggestion made by Gebhard that sadomasochism can be viewed as a theatrical performance, and the application of this perspective to the heterosexual S&M scenario by Weinberg. In fact, a unifying element in all of the papers in this collection is their emphasis upon the importance of social meanings, social control, and fantasies in the S&M world.

Thomas S. Weinberg and Gerhard Falk

The Social Organization
of Sadism and Masochism

INTRODUCTION

Sadism and masochism, the giving and receiving of pain for erotic gratification, have been largely neglected as areas for sociological study. As two
recent papers point out, descriptions of the social aspects of this behavior
are virtually nonexistent in the professional literature (Spengler, 1977;
Weinberg, 1978). The apparent lack of interest in studying sadomasochistic
behavior from a sociological perspective may be attributable to its having
been traditionally examined from a psychoanalytic model. The influence of
such writers as Krafft-Ebing (1932) and Sigmund Freud (1938) may have
been to obscure the social aspects of this behavior by defining it solely in
terms of individual pathology. Inasmuch as sociologists have until quite
recently ignored sadomasochism, descriptions of its social aspects have been
largely left to journalists (e.g., Coburn, 1977; Halpern, 1977; Smith and
Cox, 1979a and 1979b). This is unfortunate, because these journalistic
observations are neither systematic nor theoretical.

In this paper we present, in a preliminary way, some sociological observations drawn from an ongoing research project, which began in December
1977. Our focus is on the ways in which contacts are made among participants in the sadomasochistic (S&M) world, sadomasochistic organizations, and other subcultural supports for and influences upon this behavior.
We are primarily concerned with heterosexual sadomasochism, an area that
has been less examined than the homosexual S&M world. Although there
are some points of contact between these two S&M subcultures, and even

Reprinted from *Deviant Behavior: An Interdisciplinary Journal,* 1:379-393, 1980.
Reprinted by permission of the author.

though some individuals may participate in both and define their sexuality in a flexible way, the two worlds remain distinct. The homosexual S&M world is much more visible, with many large cities having at least one so-called leather bar. As Spengler (1977) has noted, only homosexual sado-masochists appear to be approachable for study. Heterosexual sado-masochists are extremely reluctant to be interviewed or studied in any way.

METHODS

Given the difficulties in contacting a large sample of sadomasochists,[1] our conclusions must remain tentative. Our data consist of a few formal and informal interviews with men engaging in S&M behavior and with prostitutes, or "dominatrixes," specializing in "female domination." Like Spengler, we found it impossible to question sadomasochistically oriented women who were not involved in prostitution. Our only information about such women comes indirectly through conversations with their husbands, who were them-selves involved in sadomasochism. Additional sources of information on the social organization of sadomasochism comes from advertisements, flyers, magazines, and literature produced by sadomasochistic organizations.

Our contacts with respondents were made through answering advertise-ments placed in S&M contact magazines. We presented ourselves as profes-sional sociologists who were interested in understanding the S&M sub-culture. Respondents generally wished to remain anonymous; they used pseudonyms and preferred to make contacts on the telephone rather than in person. Other contacts were made fortuitously through people who knew the nature of the study.[2]

SOCIOLOGICAL STUDIES OF SADOMASOCHISM

The few studies of sadism and masochism in the sociological literature point out that S&M is a well established subculture characterized by publi-cations, a market economy, and its own argot. Howard S. Becker (1963), for instance, estimated that one catalog devoted to sadomasochistic fetish-ism, which he had examined, contained between fifteen and twenty thou-sand photographs for sale; and he therefore concluded that the dealer "did a land-office business and had a very sizable clientele" (1962:20-21). Becker further emphasized the importance of some sort of sadomasochistic sub-culture in developing deviant motivations through providing people with the appropriate conceptual linguistic tools:

Deviant motivations have a social character even when most of the activity is carried on in a private, secret, and solitary fashion. In such cases, various media of communication may take the place of face-to-face interaction in inducting the individual into the culture. The pornographic pictures I mentioned earlier were described to prospective buyers in a stylized language. Ordinary words were used in a technical shorthand designed to whet specific tastes. . . . One does not acquire a taste for "bondage photos" without having learned what they are and how they may be enjoyed (Becker, 1963:31).

John Gagnon (1977) notes the existence of clubs for heterosexuals interested in sadomasochism:

The formalization of the sadomasochistic aspects of the gay community has been paralleled by the creation of "clubs" for heterosexual masochists and sadists. Such sites offer opportunities for people with common sexual preferences to meet. Where once the problems of meeting were solved through word of mouth and through advertisements of various sorts, there is now a more public "velvet underground" in various cities which offers an opportunity for more interaction, and the creation of a local sadomasochistic culture. The city in this case provides for sexual minorities what it provided for literary minorities in the past (Gagnon, 1977:329).

A questionnaire study by Andreas Spengler (1977) of sadomasochistic West German men, however, casts doubt upon the importance of sadomasochistic clubs for making sexual contacts, at least for heterosexual men. He found that these heterosexual men were not so well integrated into a sadomasochistic subculture as were bisexual and homosexual men. Fewer heterosexual men participated in sadomasochistic parties, had an acquaintance with like-minded people, or were successful in receiving responses to advertisements placed in sadomasochistic publications. Prostitution was a more important sadomasochistic outlet for heterosexual men than it was for the other respondents. Spengler explains this finding by noting that there are few (nonprostitute) women who participate in the sadomasochistic subculture. Observations of sadomasochistic clubs and parties by journalists (e.g., Halpern, 1977; Smith and Cox, 1979a) who note a heavy preponderance of men and the presence of professional dominatrixes at these functions tend to support Spengler's findings. Spengler's "unsystematic impression" is that "nearly all the subcultural groups among heterosexual sadomasochists exist in cooperation with prostitutes" (1977:455) and that one of the functions of these heterosexually oriented sadomasochistic subcultures is to maintain for their members the fiction that prostitutes are "really" passionately involved in the sadomasochistic encounter.

Thomas S. Weinberg (1978) emphasizes the importance of sadomasochistic organizations in developing and disseminating apologias, attitudes, and ideologies supportive of sadomasochism that enable their members to justify their sexual desires. He points out the importance of fantasy and theatricality in the sadomasochistic world and examines the ways in which "frameworks" and "keys," delimiting and cuing sadomasochistic episodes, are developed through the use of a shared subcultural argot.

Joann S. DeLora and Carol A. B. Warren (1977) believe that there is a general acceptance of "the milder forms of sadistic or masochistic pleasure" in American culture (1977:366), and they note the existence of "sadomasochistic games by couples as a part of their love-making rituals" (1977:267). This does not, however, necessarily mean that either sadomasochistic behavior or sadomasochistic subcultures are widespread in this society.

MAKING CONTACTS IN THE SUBCULTURE

There are a number of ways in which sadomasochistic contacts are made. These include placing or responding to advertisements in contact magazines and other publications, finding partners through participation in other subcultural settings such as bars or swingers' clubs or through participation in prostitution. Some contacts occur by chance; others develop through encounters in sadomasochistic organizations (Weinberg, 1978).

Advertisements

The most common means of reaching other S&M devotees appears to be the use of advertisements in sadomasochistic contact magazines. Spengler (1977) found that these ads were the most frequently used way of finding partners and that only 7 percent of his sample had never placed one. The advertisements contained in contact magazines are usually organized by region, with the advertiser identified only by a code number. The ads state the preferences, requirements, and so forth of their placers. Some of the ads are accompanied by photographs, purportedly of the advertisers.

Placing and Responding to Advertisements

Procedures for placing ads and responding to them are similar in all of these magazines. In order to place an ad, one submits a fee ranging from about $5 to $10 and certifies to being over the age of twenty-one. Some publications also require that advertisers subscribe to the publication at an additional cost of $10 or more. In order to respond to an ad, some magazines require that one be a subscriber or a member of a club sponsored by the publisher. Responding to an ad costs $1 to $2 per letter. The letters are placed in stamped envelopes with the advertisers' code numbers on them. All of the envelopes are then put into a larger envelope, which also contains the publisher's fee. The publisher then addresses the coded envelopes to the advertisers and thus assures their anonymity. Our experience with this process indicates that the publishers at least do forward the letters if it is at all possible and even go so far as to return undeliverable letters at their own expense. Many of the advertisers also appear to be legitimate. When we sent letters to advertisers in our region, we received responses from some of these people. However, we are still attempting to increase our sample through these informants, an obviously difficult undertaking.

Most of the ads found in S&M contact magazines are supposedly placed by women, the majority of whom are self-described "dominants." The men tend to be "submissives" (Weinberg, 1978). This appears to be the most commonly occurring combination in North American S&M culture. Part of the explanation for the large representation of female advertisers may be that women are usually not charged a fee for advertising, that many of the female advertisers are prostitutes ("Seeks very rich slaves only"; "Photos, used lingerie for sale"; "Correspondence welcome but I expect compensation for my time"), and that the purchasers of these magazines are predominantly males seeking dominant females.

According to some of our respondents, they sometimes place ads in the "personals" colums of local newspapers. These ads are disguised as inquiries for "pen pals." Since swingers also use the same kinds of ads ("Modern couple desires couples as pen pals"; "Couple, 30, desires discreet pen pals"), it is difficult to ascertain whether an ad is a swingers' advertisement or an S&M inquiry. Both use similar code words such as "modern" or "discreet" to indicate a sexual interest. Infrequently, an S&M advertiser will include a phrase such as "interested in English culture" to indicate a preference for being whipped.

Advertisements and the Communication of Fantasy

Many of the advertisements found in contact magazines illustrate a major aspect of the sadomasochistic subculture; it is, to a large degree, a fantasy world. One cannot fully understand the organization of the S&M scene unless the central importance of the expression of fantasy for its participants is recognized. The subculture serves to segregate the sexual fantasy needs of its members from other aspects of their lives. This is often accomplished by setting up a particular theatrical situation, frequently aided by props and costumes of various kinds, in which the participants don new identities and act out different parts. Popular situations include, for example, the naughty schoolboy who is reprimanded (i.e., verbally degraded) and physically punished by the female school teacher, and the patient who is given an enema by a nurse. The importance of fantasy (and its components of hostility) is apparent in the following ads drawn from contact publications:

1. Blonde Dominatrix dressed in rubber or leather costume. Seeks experienced or novice slaves who believe in Dominant Female Superiority. I'm well qualified in B&D, watersports, humiliation, petticoat training and have equipment built by slaves.

2. Tall, cruel, Creole Beauty seeks Dominant Male partner to assist her in controlling & discipling her many slaves. Come be my King so we can play King & Queen. Do not answer if you are not sincere and generous. Letter, photo & phone gets you a surprisingly quick reply. This is for dominants only, have too many slaves now.

3. Beautiful Dominatrix, 24. A true sophisticate of the bizarre and unusual. I have a well equipped dungeon in my luxurious home. You will submit to prolonged periods of degradation for my pleasure. Toilet servitude a must. I know what you crave and can fulfill your every need.

4. Very pretty 30 yr old female has fantasies about receiving hand-spankings on bare behind. I've never allowed myself to act out any of the fantasies. Is there anyone out there who'd like to correspond with me about their fantasies or experiences with spankings?

5. Cruel husband seeking experienced dominant man to assist in training petite, shy, young wife. Eager to watch her transformed from shy, personal, sex slave to slut. Presently serving me and friend in humiliation, verbal abuse, deep throat, GR., golden shower, lewd dancing, nude posing, public display. Prefer man with extensive movie/ erotica collection, over 50, obese with a fetish for petite, young girls or hung Black. Also those with aggressive Bi-partners or trained pets.

These ads, as is apparent, contain coded messages. The language of S&M serves to indicate to potential respondents the advertisers' expectations and the sorts of roles and relationships they are looking for. For example, "B&D" (Bondage and Discipline) refers to tying up or restraining a person, along with the possibility of some sort of physical punishment. "Watersports" refers to urination. "Petticoat training" indicates cross-dressing. "Toilet servitude" (or, sometimes, "toilet training") refers to the handling of feces, being defecated upon, or to coprophagia. The abbreviation "GR" stands for "Greek," an indication that the advertiser is interested in anal intercourse. "Golden shower" is code for being urinated upon, sometimes with the inclusion of urolagnia.*

Participation in the sadomasochistic subculture also often develops out

---

*coprophagia refers to the ingestion of feces; urolagnia is the ingestion of urine—*Eds.*

of contacts made in other "deviant" sexual scenes, such as the swinging sub-culture, gay bars, and prostitution. Interestingly, some of the same people who advertise in the S&M contact magazines of one publisher also advertise in the swinging publications of another, using the same picture but with a somewhat different advertisement.

Prostitution and S&M Contacts

Prostitution is an important source of sexual contacts for sadomasochis-tically oriented men (DeLora and Warren, 1977; Spengler, 1977; Weinberg, 1978). Prostitutes have written autobiographical descriptions of their parti-cipation in this behavior (Hollander, 1972; Von Cleef, 1974). Many profes-sional dominatrixes advertise not only in sadomasochistic contact publica-tions, but also in sex-oriented publications such as *Screw*. Our interviews with professional prostitutes who specialize in "Houses of Domination" indicate a highly developed skill in S&M. Prostitutes with whom we have spoken pointed out that specializing in sadomasochism is far more lucrative than conventional prostitution.[3] Fees range from $35 to $45 for half an hour, and from $50 to $100 or more for an hour's session. A number of prostitutes advertise "No Straight Sex, S&M and TV (i.e., transvestitism) only" and do not, they claim, have sexual intercourse with their clientele. Apart from the development of special skills and the creation of fantasy scenarios, professional dominatrixes appear to differ little from women engaged in conventional prostitution. Like the more usual forms of prosti-tution, sadomasochistic specialists practice their trade in houses of prosti-tution, massage parlors (*Evening Tribune,* 1980), and as individual entrepreneurs.

Chance Contacts

Some contacts are made accidentally. One respondent told us, for example, that he was approached and engaged in conversation by a number of men who were attracted by his wife's leather coat and high leather boots, although she had not purposely worn them to advertise her interest in S&M. One way to encourage such approaches, then, is to display symbols com-monly accepted in the sadomasochistic subculture. This does not appear to be a very common practice among heterosexual devotees of S&M, apart from their participation in S&M parties, although participants in the homosexual leather scene frequently wear symbols such as colored handker-chiefs or strategically located key chains to advertise their preferences.

Initial Meetings: Determining Compatibility

When contacts are first made among sadomasochists, they follow a format similar to the initial sizing up that occurs among swingers (Bartell, 1971; Palson and Palson, 1972). This is not surprising; some informants have told us that they were introduced to sadomasochism through swinging. Typically, two couples may go out to dinner and spend relatively little time discussing their sexuality. Rather, the purpose of their meeting is to discover, in a non-threatening situation, whether they are comfortable with each other and socially compatible. One respondent who is a business executive noted that social compatibility is important because sexual activity takes up a relatively small amount of an evening's time and "you have to have something to talk about with the other couple." His group consists of other professionals, such as dentists and attorneys.

Since the S&M scene demands absolute trust and confidence in another person, especially if one may be bound helplessly and gagged, this initial meeting is a critical one. Only after people have built up a certain amount of trust do they proceed to engage in sadomasochistic activities.

Before an actual scene occurs, the participants in it discuss their needs, fantasies, fears, and what they are and are not willing to do. What ultimately occurs during a scene is the outcome of this discussion, in which the original thoughts are somewhat modified, then subjected to a bargaining process by which the verbalized desires of the partner are accommodated. This accommodation appears to be necessary because the participants wish to carry their imagination into action by convincing their partner that their wishes are reasonably compatible. Unless there is agreement, there probably will not be mutual gratification. Contrary to the popular notion that the sadist is in command of this situation, S&M devotees often assert that it is the masochist who controls the scene, because it is his or her fantasies that the sadist acts out.

S&M ORGANIZATIONS AND THEIR FUNCTIONS

There are a number of formally organized sadomasochistic clubs and numerous informal groups of sadists and masochists throughout this country. For the purpose of this discussion, we will classify them roughly into the following categories, based upon what seem to be their primary activities: (1) discussion or consciousness-raising groups, (2) publishing organizations, (3) sex clubs, and (4) theatrical companies.[4]

Discussion or Consciousness-raising Groups

The Till Eulenspiegel Society[5] in New York City describes itself as a "discussion and consciousness-raising group," the objective of which is "to promote better understanding and self-awareness of these (sadomasochistic) drives so that they may be enjoyed as a part of a full sex life, rather than set aside out of fear or guilt." The society explicitly denies being "in any sense a sex club or swingers' organization." During the Eulenspiegel's weekly meetings, members discuss their feelings and behavior and occasionally are given demonstrations and lectures by sadomasochistic experts. Although Eulenspiegel does not appear to propagandize to the larger society nor to lobby for legal change, it does seem to resemble in some of its avowed purposes other minority organizations, such as those studied by Yearwood and Weinberg (1979). Despite the Eulenspiegel Society's denial that it is a sex club, it does, in fact, sponsor parties at which sadomasochistic behavior occurs (Halpern, 1977).

Publishing Organizations

The House of Milan, located in Los Angeles, publishes a number of contact magazines (*Latent Image, Aggressive Gals, Bitch Goddesses*) that serve to facilitate communication among S&M devotees throughout the country. They also publish magazines for those who enjoy simply reading about female domination, spanking, transvestism, rubber fetishes, and so on. This organization gives parties occasionally, which are advertised in its contact publications.

I. Dictor Enterprises in Philadelphia publishes a sadomasochistic contact magazine called *Amazon*. The aim of this magazine, according to its former publisher, Malibu Publications, is to "provide the average person with a publication that reveals S&M/B&D as a normal form of sexual activity and alleviates any feelings of guilt and/or perversion arising from long held misconceptions." To this end, the magazine includes not only contact ads, but also a question and answer column written by "a clinical psychologist with a long, widely varied experience in sex therapy and family counseling"; a section containing news about new publications, other organizations, films of interest to S&M devotees, sources of products; news of upcoming events and the like; fiction involving sadomasochistic interests and behavior; cartoons; and commercial advertisements for other clubs, films, and sexual devices.

Sex Clubs

Chateau 19 is an "on-premise S&M club" (Smith and Cox, 1979a) in New York City. Its twice-weekly sessions are open to the public. For an admission fee ($7.50 for men, $2.50 for women, including two drinks) one is free to participate in any of the night's activities. Smith and Cox (1979a) reported that there was a wide range in the ages of the club's habitues, with most being between the ages of twenty-five and thirty-five. From their description, Chateau 19 appears to be very similar to other on-premise, impersonal sex clubs such as Plato's Retreat in New York City, San Francisco's Sutro Bath House, and gay baths found throughout the country.

Theatrical Companies

Sadomasochistic fantasies have been brought "out of the closet" by an organization known as "The Project." The Project, which calls itself a "research team," was founded in the early 1970s by a New York City radio personality. It has been featured on talk shows on the three major television networks and has been written about in a number of popular culture and sexually oriented newspapers and magazines. Performers in The Project travel throughout the state to churches, colleges, singles groups, private parties, and various social organizations, acting out for a fee, fantasies that they have collected through "hundreds of interviews and thousands of letters." The program of one of their productions, called "Another Way to Love," included the following S&M scenarios:[6]

1. "'The Beauty of Looking Beastly': An authentic psychosexual fairy tale wherein the 'ugliest man in the world' lives his most beautiful moment" (a scene in which a man is publicly humiliated by a beautiful woman who forces him to wear a collar and leash and a mask hiding his face).
2. "'I'm the Haughtiest Girl in the Whole USA': Wherein a fetishistic 'judge' who specializes in 'justice' for pretty girls convicted of pretty-girl crimes liquifies his toughest prisoner into a splash pool of humiliation by getting to the bottom of her evil" (a scene in which a man dressed as a monk puts a woman into stocks, forcing her to publicly confess her crime of "haughtiness," and then tortures her by tickling her bare feet).
3. "'Bottoms Up!': A peek into the bedroom of an earnest young wife who endeavors to redesign her color scheme by pestering, plaguing, and provoking her posterior decorator" (a spanking fantasy).
4. "'Paul(a)': Wherein the fantasist awakens her husband to a galaxy of life changes most profound" (a scene in which a woman, dressed in a translucent black body suit, high heeled boots, and armed with a whip, forces her husband to dress up in a French maid's uniform, complete with female undergarments and a wig).

The list of organizations described above is in no sense exhaustive;

however, it does serve to illustrate the variety of more formally developed associations found within the sadomasochistic subculture. Although the purposes of these organizations appear to vary widely, from enterprises designed to make a profit for their owners to those, like Eulenspiegel, that exist to help sadomasochists accept their inclinations, they nevertheless serve similar functions for persons interested in S&M. First, they all provide the possibilities of sexual outlets, either through direct participation as in Chateau 19 or in the parties given by other organizations, through the opportunity to make connections with similarly inclined people by advertising in contact magazines such as *Amazon,* or through the use of these magazines to stimulate sexual fantasies. Second, all of these organizations serve to disseminate information about sadomasochism to their members, enabling the latter to learn new techniques, develop new interests, and find out about events, news, and so forth relevant to their needs. Third, all of the sadomasochistic organizations develop and communicate, either explicitly or implicitly, justifications and apologias enabling people to accept their feelings and behavior as perfectly normal. Fourth, by providing these special settings, justifications, and the appropriate linguistic tools, they enable people to segregate their sadomasochistic needs and behavior from other areas of their lives.

CONCLUSIONS

Although sadomasochism has traditionally been studied as an individual psychopathology, in many instances this behavior is a group phenomenon. A variety of sadomasochistic groups and organizations facilitate contacts among members, teach new techniques and behaviors, and serve to normalize individuals' attitudes, interests, and sexual activities. A more comprehensive understanding of sadomasochism requires that it be examined within a broader social context, rather than remain limited to a study of individual case histories. When this is done, some alternative ways of thinking about sadomasochism emerge. For example, S&M may serve recreational as well as sexual needs for its devotees. One journalist (Coburn, 1977:45) speculates that a new sort of S&M "chic" has been developing in this country, and she cites recent popular magazine articles, popular music, billboard advertisements, and so forth, all with S&M motifs as evidence for this speculation. Sadomasochistic themes also appear in recent movies (e.g., *Myra Breckenridge, The Opening of Misty Beethoven,* and *Wholly Moses!* among others) and in novels. Another way of looking at sadomasochism is in terms of economics. Sadomasochistic publications are filled with ads from manufacturers of expensive wearing apparel, devices, equipment, and so forth. There seems to be a lucrative business in magazines, movies, sex clubs, prostitution, and the like, all aimed at a sadomasochistic market.

NOTES

1. Spengler (1977:442) acknowledges this problem when he states, "Extreme difficulties exist in questioning sadomasochists. Heterosexual sadomasochists live undercover; their groups are cut off from the outside world. . . . Anonymity is one of the special norms of sadomasochistic subcultures."

2. One such chance contact occurred when one of the writers happened to casually mention the study to a former student whom he met one day in the student union. A few hours later, he was surprised by a telephone call from this man, who told him that he had spoken to a friend who might be interested in discussing sadomasochism. About an hour later, the writer received a call from his student's friend, a young woman who had been a prostitute, a dominatrix, and a madame in a house of female domination. Over a lengthy lunch the next day, this woman and the writer discussed his work in sadomasochism. She was particularly concerned about his personal reasons for the study (was he really a policeman, or a voyeur, or a sadomasochist attempting to use the research for his own sexual purposes?) and spent the time probing his motivations. Apparently convinced that he had no ulterior motives, understood people in deviant lifestyles, and could be trusted, she became an invaluable resource for contacts and information about the S&M world.

3. Some quotations from our interviews with dominatrixes are reproduced elsewhere (Weinberg, 1978: especially pp. 286-287). The transcript of a fascinating interview with a professional prostitute specializing in S&M appears in Smith and Cox (1979b).

4. There are, of course, any number of ways in which these organizations could be classified, such as according to whether they are profit or non-profit enterprises, whether they serve to facilitate sexual contacts and in what specific ways they do this, whether they are politically oriented and so on.

5. The organization takes its name from a figure in German folklore who is said to have carried heavy loads up mountains because it felt so good when he put these burdens down and thus acknowledged his presumably masochistic tendencies.

6. The writers first became aware of the existence of The Project when one of them saw an advertisement for one of its productions in a Buffalo, New York, homophile publication. He attended the performance, which was held in the Buffalo Gay Community Services Center, in March 1976. The show consisted of a half-dozen scenarios, four of which are described above, performed by a male and a female actor. This was followed by a discussion period, during which the audience could ask the actors questions. In addition to its prerehearsed shows,

The Project also acts out individuals' private fantasies at its own location in New York City. The individual, who pays a fee for this service, does not participate in the performance of his own fantasy, however, but remains strictly an observer. The Project does not appear to have been conceived solely as a profit-making venture for its creator, however. At the conclusion of its two Buffalo performances, the actors made a donation of several hundred dollars to support the activities of the Gay Center. Considering the low cost of admission to the performances ($3 for a Sunday matinee and $3.50 for that evening's show), the fairly small attendance, and travel expenses, The Project does not seem to have made very much money during its visit.

REFERENCES

Bartell, Gilbert D. 1971, *Group Sex.* New York: Signet Books.

Becker, Howard S. 1963, *Outsiders: Studies in the Sociology of Deviance.* New York: Free Press.

Coburn, Judith 1977, "S&M" *New Times* 8 (Feb. 4): 43–50.

DeLora, Joann S., and Carol A. B. Warren 1977, *Understanding Sexual Interaction.* Boston: Houghton-Mifflin.

Evening Tribune (San Diego) 1980, "Parlor operator sentenced." (Jan. 23): B-6.

Freud, Sigmund 1938, *The Basic Writings of Sigmund Freud.* (A. A. Brill, trans. and ed.). New York: Modern Library.

Gagnon, John 1977, *Human Sexualities.* Glenview, Ill.: Scott, Foresman.

Halpern, Bruce 1977, "Spanks for the memory." *Screw* 420 (March 21): 4–7.

Hollander, Xaviera 1972, *The Happy Hooker.* New York: Dell.

Krafft-Ebing, R. von. 1932, *Psychopathia Sexualis.* New York: Physicians' and Surgeons' Book Company.

Palson, Charles and Rebecca Palson 1972, "Swinging in wedlock." *Transaction/Society* 9 (Feb.): 28–37.

Smith, Howard and Cathy Cox 1979a, "Scenes: s&m in the open." *Village Voice* 24 (Jan. 15): 24. 1979b, "Scenes: dialogue with a dominatrix." *Village Voice* 24 (Jan. 29): 19–20.

Spengler, Andreas 1977, "Manifest sadomasochism of males: results of an empirical study." *Archives of Sexual Behavior* 6: 441–56.

Von Cleef, Monique 1971, *The House of Pain,* Secaucus, N.J.: Lyle Stuart.

Weinberg, Thomas S. 1978, "Sadism and masochism: sociological perspectives." *Bulletin of the American Academy of Psychiatry and the Law* 6: 284–95.

Yearwood, Lennox and Thomas S. Weinberg 1979, "Black organizations, gay organizations: sociological parallels," pp. 301–16 in Martin P. Levine (ed.), *Gay Men: The Sociology of Male Homosexuality.* New York: Harper and Row.

G. W. Levi Kamel

Leathersex: Meaningful Aspects of Gay Sadomasochism

DATA AND METHODS

Leathersex is visible for the social sciences by way of adult literature and homosexual meeting places. My own employ in an adult bookstore led to innumerable opportunities for exposure to S&M people. Leathersex publications were scrutinized regularly, and periodic analysis of related pornographic novels and photos helped to confirm findings. Sex ads pertaining to S&M were analyzed from prior research (Laner and Kamel, 1977). When sufficient rapport could be established with regular bookstore customers, heterosexual and homosexual, taped interviews were conducted. Three years of conversational interaction in leather-oriented bars across the United States and Europe created an invaluable overall impression of leathersex. But the bulk of information for this research is the result of informal conversations while in the role of potential participant, an insider role genuinely expected of the newcomer by experienced leathermen.[1]

ACTION: THE PRACTICES OF THE LEATHERMEN

For leathermen, S&M refers to the desire for dominance and submission. Acting out impulses to dominate or submit is accomplished by any number of practices. Most activities revolve around four basics: restraint, humiliation, masculinity, and fear. These feelings as they apply to the leathermen

A revised version of an article which appears in *Deviant Behavior: An Interdisciplinary Journal*, 1:171–191, 1980. Reprinted by permission of the author.

are best considered from the gay sadomasochist's meanings of "masculine"/ "feminine" and "dominance"/"submission."

Leathermen see gay sex as all-male encounters, and S&M for them is the ultimate in man-to-man interaction. In our culture, we understand dominance as masculine and submission as feminine, without the need to qualify such terms. But among leathermen, submission is not equated with feminine; "male submission" and the feeling of "masculine submissiveness" are, for them, perceptions with no contradiction. With this in mind, it is likely that gay masochists have fewer identity difficulties than their straight counterparts. The heterosexual masochist represents a cultural contradiction—he is masculine, yet submissive to women. Unlike his gay counterpart, he usually finds the task of redefining masculinity impossible. The gay man, if only because of his homosexuality, has already redefined masculinity. He does not necessarily "lose his maleness," or "wish to be a woman." Rather, maleness is understood not always in terms of dominance; it can be submissive, too.

In an aura of masculinity, then, the S (master or sadist) will dominate, and the M (slave or masochist) is willfully dominated. Even though basically an illusion, a game, the S&M scene[2] is most satisfying for participants when these emotional desires are acted out. Again, the activities and desires most consistently mentioned during interviews and informal discussions; in literature, publications, and pornography; and in the content of the sex ads reveal the four basic themes of restraint via bondage; humiliation via language, physical degradation, and watersports; masculinity via leather and roughness; and fear via threat of violence and pain. Though by no means exhaustive, these themes are central to the interests and activities of the gay sadomasochist.

Restraint: Role Establishment

Bondage, or restraint, achieved through the use of ropes, leather devices of all sorts, chains, or even heavy equipment such as racks and stretchers, is often employed during a scene—often at the very beginning. A few U.S. and European cities have gay S&M bathhouse setups with every imaginable restraining device available, from simple finger cuffs to a sophisticated reproduction of the French guillotine. Bondage, as used in the S&M scene, serves to establish roles, to deprive the slave of his choice of activities, and to direct power to the master. As symbolized by restraint, the slave yields his freedom to another man.

Bondage may be found as a scene in itself and will take on different meanings when not used in an S&M relationship. Likewise, S&M is sufficiently independent of bondage that leathersex may proceed without physical restraints. In this case, according to Larry Townsend's *The Leatherman's Handbook* (1977:66):

> S&M without bondage is the M's (the slave's) game . . . we deal here with the possibility of his moving out of the encounter if it ceases to turn him on. For this reason, the S (master) is faced with an even more difficult task. He is deprived of full physical control, and must maintain his command by other than ropes, or chains, or straps.

Fantasy thus becomes the primary device restraining the slave, and he is made to feel that any attempt to leave the presence of his master would be in vain, and would only elicit more punishment. The M will usually test the validity of his restraint, and at the same time verify his imprisonment in order to maintain his fantasy. And in response to attempted escapes, the S will more firmly establish his dominance by way of activities that humiliate, "demasculate,"[3] or inculcate fear. With or without the ropes, physical or psychological restraints help to establish and maintain roles.

Humiliation: Role Performance

Humiliation is a key ingredient in most S&M scenes. Although humiliation may have certain meanings for sexual scenes outside of S&M, for leathermen it is the method by which they carry out their respective roles. In this sense, masochists are in the act of being slaves and sadists are being masters, when performing acts of humiliation.

The master uses many methods to humble his slave, but among the most commonly employed is verbal humiliation, which involves the use of degrading name-calling (e.g., "cocksucker," "punk," and "worthless slut"). In addition, verbal activity includes dispensing of harsh-sounding commands and using terms or phrases that threaten the slave's well-being. According to several experienced leathermen, not all degrading terms are erotic. It may take several encounters and discussions before the S will hit upon a "magic word" for his M.

> I finally figured out after two years with Frank that he loves to be called a "punk-sucker." I stand over him with Levis on, pinch his neck to let him know who's boss, and say, "Pull it out, punk-sucker." Now he comes before I do.

Verbal interaction, designed to demean the M and give the S a chance to use his authority, may be essential to an encounter. This can be illustrated in the following verbal construct:

S: Beg for it, slave.
M: Please let me have it.
S: Please what, you asshole.
M: Please, sir!
S: You'll get it, when I'm ready.
M: Please, sir, now.
S: Maybe I'll whip you first.

Derogatory names, commands, and threats of violence are all directed toward the M, in an attempt to satisfy his desire to be humiliated.

Another strain of degradation, less common than verbal abuse, is "kennel discipline," or demasculation and dehumanization of the M by treating him literally like a dog. Licking the master's boots, being led around on a leash, wearing a dog collar, and even being forced to eat from a dog bowl are all possibilities. In more involved relationships, the slave may even spend an occasional night at the foot of his master's bed. Kennel discipline can become so involved that it may, on rare occasions, carry over to nonsexual parts of a relationship. This is an example of what Weinberg, following Goffman, has referred as "breaking frame," in a previous essay in this volume.

Watersports, the use of urination during sexual activity, is most often thought of as a sexual variance for its own sake, and indeed it commonly is (Ellis, 1966:87). But when applied to S&M, its purpose is to degrade the slave and "exalt" the master. The difference in meaning is that in the former use of watersports, there is erotic fascination with the sight of urination itself, with or without the desire to come into contact. But in the latter, the S&M scene, being urinated on becomes symbolic of being degraded, used, and worthless. Actually, many of the usual watersports activities that entail extensive setups and cleanup: scatology, enemas, and other "bathroom sex," pose a problem in S&M — that of breaking the established mood. For urination, mats, bathtubs, and enclosed back yards are most practical, since such settings are easily moved into and out of.

Masculinity: Role Definition

Leather articles are essential to some, of some importance to others, and of no importance to still others involved in leathersex.[4] Leather is, of course, a popular fetish in itself, but with S&M it can be a strong symbol of masculinity. More specifically, leather represents the outward manifestation of "butchness," roughness, and the macho image. It is most often black leather that is approved of in the social or sexual settings of the leathermen.

For some men, it is the look of leather that makes it appealing, especially when worn by an attractive man. Others like the taste of leather. Still others are aroused by the feel of it—usually, but not always, when someone is in it. The degree of importance of black leather is extremely situational and may depend on what the leather object is, who one's partner is, and how that item is used. The most common articles of leather are cockrings (straps of leather that in some way constrain the genitals), jockstraps, belts, boots, whips, and straps (for restraint, to threaten violence, or to wear with metal rings), jackets, and mats, to name a few. Steel is less commonly used than leather articles and usually takes the form of studs, spike inlays in leather, or retraints, such as handcuffs or wrist and ankle clamps.[5]

Human sexual feelings are such that interpretation and speculation on the meanings of specific acts by individuals are open to a great many possibilities. To illustrate, consider an isolated event during an all-male sexual encounter. A masculine man clad in tight leather pants, stands macho-style over his slave; and, on command, the slave begins licking his master's crotch. A researcher stumbles upon the scene. Having been exposed to a diversity of lifestyles, he has a basic understanding of what he is observing; that is, he sees two men in an act of sexual expression. In lieu of running off in shock at the sight, he decides that his researcher's curiosity is piqued more than his heterosexuality is offended. He therefore remains hidden and, pulling out the pen and pad he carries, he notes an immediately observable phenomenon: Both men have erections. He interprets this, quite accurately, as an indication that both men are sexually aroused by this single act (i.e., one man licking the black, leather-clad genitals of another). At this point, our observer becomes aroused also, in an intellectual sense, and asks Why? From the standpoint of his own sexuality, the observer is not nearly so puzzled by the master's turgid state as he is by the slave's. The observer decides to explore possible explanations.

First, it may be that the slave is aroused only because he was commanded to do the act. His excitement is due to a commanding voice, not the act itself, not the leather, and perhaps not even his master. Further, he could have been commanded to do any number of things, and the result would have been the same, as long as he defined the command in an erotic way. Second, perhaps the arousal is due to the act of licking in the area of another man's genitals, with the hope of eventual contact. The leather is not only irrelevant, but a nuisance, and the command is only tolerable if he eventually gets what he wants most. A third possibility is that our slave is turned on because the leather he is licking is his master's leather. Without regard for what his S has on, he is still aroused by the clothes that represent his master's authority, dominance, and masculinity. Further, anyone in the same clothes who did not "own" him would not be as attractive. A fourth possibility is that for the slave the leather is a full-blown fetish, and in sexually defined situations such as this, it is the taste, smell, feel, or all three sensations that thrill him. He must prefer that someone be in the leather, but male or female, dominant or submissive, is not important. Yet another possibility is that the licking behavior itself makes him feel "like a dog," and no force, command, leather, or particular partner would affect his state of arousal. In this instance, it is his own activity that turns him on, most probably with the aid of fantasy.

Our researcher begins to realize that there is no end to the number of possible interpretations.[6] Only a candid question and answer period involving considerable rapport could reveal the meanings the slave finds in his own behavior. And even then, the interpretation would rely on the assumption that the slave is adequately in touch with his own feelings and desires.[7]

Fear: Role Maintenance

After an analytical look at sadomasochism among homosexuals, one is left with the impression that it is not born of a confusion of pain and pleasure, but rather of a redefinition of pain.[8] A sadist generally does not take pleasure in causing pain for the mere sake of the act. Nor is it pleasurable if his lover does not share the S&M definition of pain (Mass, 1979). Likewise, the masochist who stubs his toe on an unruly sidewalk does not get an erotic charge. Painful accidents are painful, with no confusion whatsoever. The pain of S&M is defined differently because it is a method by which partners maintain their dominant and submissive roles. It is a means to an end.

The whip, for example, takes on a threatening meaning for the masochist, and when in the possession of the master, it signifies who is boss. Even if used only lightly, the feel of the whip verifies or maintains their respective roles. The administration of pain is not defined as doing harm to another, but as dominating another. How much pain is desirable or tolerable is a highly individual matter, but it seems to be far less than is commonly supposed.

The means by which pain is given varies, but one of the most common methods is spanking, or more precisely, "ass slapping." Arm locks, head holds, and the like are also common. Another example is that of the S who will place a lighted candle at the proper angle for his slave to receive its drippings, sometimes while blindfolded. Generally, as an activity becomes more extreme, it is practiced and mentioned less frequently until it dwindles into the realm of fantasy.[9]

One experienced M, in a discussion on pain, explained, "The skilled master is not one who knows how to give pain, so much as he is able to inculcate the fear and the threat of pain and violence." Extremes, of course, exist. By far, most gay men in leather are not interested in, and are indeed very cautious of, extreme behavior in their sexual encounters. More than other groups, they are aware of the potential dangers of S&M. Compulsive sadists and masochists, rare as they are, may have lessened the credibility of leathersex; and the ways in which such persons are exposed and excluded are among the next set of considerations.

NORMS: THE MORES OF THE LEATHERMEN

The activities and emotions described above are those of a minority of persons, and the participants are as much aware of that fact as anyone. One result of this awareness is a group cohesiveness of sufficient strength to generate shared norms, which may be subdivided into contact norms, action norms, and relationship norms. These norms act to control membership, activities, and emotions in ways that are different from mainstream gay society. If it is the differentness of S&M norms that makes leathersex so misunderstood, then a discussion of these may clear up some misconceptions.

Contact Norms: Membership Control

While mainstream gays often shun leathermen out of fear, S&M men exclude certain groups themselves, out of a fear more justified. Although compulsive S&M types are rare and are not likely to be part of the bar scene, in the bathhouses, or responding to sex ads in underground newspapers, they nevertheless pose a real threat to leather society. One precaution is the avoidance of those who have no social recognition; thus, transients and strangers are avoided. Whereas most gays would be attracted to new faces in their midst, S&M men are more cautious. The street pickups, often found in larger cities, are less inviting for the leathermen than for most gay people; thus, hustlers are avoided. (An exception to the "no hustlers" norm may be among those masochists who answer massage ads in underground publications. But the "masseur" is presumed safer than the street hustler.) Finally, rumor of one extreme activity by an S and his reputation can quickly be ruined in a city, since those who violate known limits are avoided.[10]

A conversation with a new S&M contact may sound like a "stability test," rather than the usual small talk of most gay bar settings. The leatherman is generally more careful than his gay brothers about who he invites home. One interview with a young M revealed typical stability questions directed toward potential partners:

My conversation with someone new sometimes sounds like a questionnaire. I find out social standing, how long he's lived here, what sort of work he does, if he knows any of my friends, how much he travels, and on and on. If he has nothing to lose by violating my limits, I leave him immediately.

Implicit here is the belief that the maintenance of good social standing is valued enough to ensure safety. Social standing is equated with stability. This serves as an excellent example of the belief in the strength of informal social controls in a setting where formal controls are nonexistent. By comparison, the brand of sadomasochism often found in straight society, such as forced sex, lacks self-imposed, informal social norms for its containment. It appears to have little membership or organization. Without benefit of mutual consent, regular meeting places, or notions of limits, straight S&M often surfaces for public view in cases of violent sexual acts, usually involving unwilling victims of physical force. The social control is formal—the police departments, courts, and hospitals. Further, the S&M actions of gay men are carried out in prescribed manners, whereas action norms are rare among heterosexuals.[11]

Action Norms: Activity Control

A visit to a large city leather bar would quickly reveal to an observer that the gay S&M scene is socially, as well as sexually, laden with symbolism. The leatherman's appearance will tell his story. More than other gays, the men in leather have a lot to say about their sexual leanings, and they are inclined to say it with what they wear (Fischer, 1977).

Masters and slaves are most likely to wear Levis or leather pants, with the master more commonly in the latter. Based on their appearance, they might be compared to bikers and jocks in one bar; both of masculine image, but one more so than the other.[12] The slave often wears a hankie in his right pocket, the master's in the left. In parts of the East, the opposite is true. Although codes vary and are subject to fad, certain colors of hankies symbolize particular desires, and several hankies in one pocket can read like a porno book. One could, according to one standardized code list, expect to find some combination of the following preferences in a given leather bar: burgundy—bondage; yellow—watersports; light blue—oral preferences; dark blue—anal preferences; red—fist fucking; black—heavy S&M; orange —"anything goes." These more precise symbols are likely to be found in larger cities and only in leather bars. Many gay people would be no more familiar than Mrs. Jones with such color symbols, except to understand the meaning of which pocket is used and the more popular blue hankies. Another understanding of the subculture is the dangling of keys from one's belt on the right or left; this means passive or dominant, respectively.

Black leather jackets and motorcycle boots are almost standard, but anything in brown leather is often considered poor taste. Some slaves wear leather collars, plain or studded. Other gadgets, like handcuffs, may be worn from black, leather-studded belts to signify desires. Such a description as this is far from exhaustive, and only those totally involved in the scene could keep pace with the constant local, national, or even international changes and modifications.

Perhaps the most important of the action norms is the setting of limits, which is simply a determination of how far a person goes in a scene — what he likes and dislikes. The more experienced leathermen can accomplish this in initial bar contact conversations without destroying the mood of excitement and anticipation. The M introduces his limits in subtle or indirect ways, perhaps by briefly discussing past experiences he has enjoyed most. It is commonly the M who steers the sexual content of the conversation; in that way he prescribes the action. The wise S avoids statements that might commit him to activities that are beyond the limits of the M. If at some point the M refers to his new bar friend as "sir," it means more than submission; it issues approval and signifies acceptance. Then the S is free to respond in degrading terms to begin mood establishment, but typically not before. The intensity of erotic interaction increases when the S begins to tell the M what he will "force" him to do, but only after the slave has indicated the extent and extremes of his desires. Many gays have objected to this form of conversation on the grounds that such what-do-you-like-to-do interaction seems inappropriate to a meaningful sexual encounter. Possibly the real distaste for verbal exchange of this type is rooted in the fear that it makes gay sex essentially different from straight sex, since heterosexuals supposedly know who will do what to whom. But for those involved in leathersex, initial conversations of this sort add to — in fact, they often initiate — the erotic mood, and in effect the participants begin to have sex before leaving the bar. And again, initial discussion of preferences is necessary for the leathermen because the nature of their orientation yields a more diverse set of sexual possibilities. But while other gays avoid the what-do-you-like-to-do syndrome, the leathermen stay clear of direct or overt discussion of their tastes, lest they defeat the initial purpose of initiating eroticism.

Another key norm also used as a safety device during leathersex is the "time-out" period, which gives both men a rest, or is called when the action gets too rough. Both men have the right, by the use of subtle clues, to call time-out. For the M, time-out may be indicated by referring to his master's first name, or some other taboo behavior. The S might simply state that he will "grant" his slave a rest, when he himself wants a break. Any mutually acceptable verbal or physical sign suffices; but again, neither man wants to break the mood of dominance and submission, so low-key activities or verbal abuse may continue, replacing the heavier action. Most time-out signals take the form of behavior that *slightly* disrupts the established S&M mood.

Most masters claim for themselves the ability to distinguish a real "no" from one that means "yes" by the voice inflection. As one recalls, "A few times (my slave) has yelled 'no' loud enough for the neighbors to hear. . . . I usually get the message." And another S: "I can tell a real 'no' because the others sound fake. There's no 'no' like a real 'no'!"

One more specific S explains the difference this way: "The fake 'no' sounds more like a whine or a plea, combined with a facial look of agony. The real 'no' sounds serious, and the look is that of anger." I suspect, however, that masochists may accompany their real "no" with slight verbal mood disrupters, similar to those used to request time-out.

It is also interesting to note a norm of avoiding the authentic verbal abuses—those terms of a hostile heterosexual society—such as "queer," "fag," or "swish." Dominance and submission for most leathermen is not so real that they lose sight of a more genuine mutual respect. Likewise, their sense of self-esteem remains intact, unharmed by their activities. Outside the sexual context, an M can still be hurt in a genuine way, and an insensitive S can still be hurtful of feelings.

The literature and interviews reveal that although role exchanges during an encounter are rare, because they disrupt the S&M mood, the most exciting S has also served as an M, and the best M is capable of the S role. It is common for an S to have once been an M almost exclusively, and most leathermen begin their sexual lives as slaves. The high degree of role exchanges (even with the tendency for M role preferences in general[13]) may make S&M partners more sensitive to each other's emotional, as well as sexual, needs. In fact, other norms, involving the way in which an S and an M relate to each other in non-S&M situations, are found to exist on another level. These are, for lack of a more precise term, the interpersonal mores of the leathermen.

Relationship Norms: Emotional Control

Perhaps the most surprising revelation about S&M sex is that many times it culminates in masculine gentleness, warmth, and affection. Interviews and most scene descriptions in literature support the norm of showing intimacy for one's partner after orgasm, which serves to give the encounter deeper meaning and gratification. One man used these words to describe his long-term relationship: "(He) has the rare ability to satisfy my need to be loved, and (my) desire to submit at the same instant. One without the other is incomplete. I have always equated the two feelings in fact, and never enjoy settling for less."

Unlike the "quickie" encounters for which some gay men are notorious, total S&M scenes take more time, by the complexity of the activities. They require more than the usual commitment and trust on the part of the participants. Much more sensitivity to the feelings of one's partner is needed, and leathersex demands by its very nature a more intimate knowledge of the other man. In light of these impressions, then, perhaps it is not so shocking that leathermen express "softer," non-S&M feelings during and after an encounter.

Related to the usual higher degree of intimacy is the interesting aspect of lover arrangements among leathermen. Discussions indicate that roles often break down completely in domestic affairs. There is little relationship between sex role and daily duties (Townsend, 1977). S&M is viewed as a fulfilling game, one not always needed or desired, and usually not central to the relationship. The general gay objection to S&M sex as "only a scene" is not grounded in the fact that the term *scene* is redefined by S&M men as a "desirable encounter"; it is only a game perhaps, but one that is meaningful for those involved.

Men of the leather scene may be better able to express physical attraction without confusing it with love. The leathermen will more likely recognize each other's presence when they meet in bars, even when sexual attraction has worn off. They seem well equipped to express the precise feelings they retain for each other and are less likely to keep each other guessing about the "meaning" of past sexual encounters. They appear free to exhibit emotion without conventional obligation.

Among serious lovers, the positive S&M relationship is seen as a "total relationship," a unit of complementary desires. The master and slave are two sides of the same coin and fuse to the extent that the term "role" is only a convenient label, meaningless in reality. The world of male homosexuals is often depicted as one of an endless procession of acts of sex, with little concern for person, location, or emotion. True or not, such a view does not seem applicable to S&M relationships. They appear to be among the most stable arrangements of the gay community, bound by considerable emotional and personal investment, and not simply by ropes.

NOTES

1. While talking to leathermen in the adult book stores and in S&M bars of major U.S. and European cities, I expressed interest in the scene on a personal level and overheard usual public bar conversation. Within all-male cruise bars, terminating interaction is generally easier than it is in most other settings, so that I found no difficulty separating intellectual interest from personal intention.

2. There are two reasons why the word "scene" is applicable in reference to gay S&M activities. First, it is used by the participants themselves. Second, its use should suggest that these activities may be analyzed as a theatrical performance without loss of empirical grounding. This work is intended to be more closely tied to the development of existential sociology with an emphasis on the link between private meaning and the emergence of a scene.

3. An analysis of pornography suggests that demasculation among heterosexual sadomasochists means 'feminizing,' usually through forced

cross-dressing. Among homosexuals it means being dominated by another man *as* a man and cross-dressing is rarely involved. Cross-dressing would destroy the entire meaning of the scene.

4. The term "leathersex" is used in place of S&M in serious books and publications (as opposed to pornography), but is not often used among gays themselves, except perhaps by the most experienced. While leather is strongly equated with S&M among both heterosexuals and homosexuals, it is not a necessary ingredient.

5. Most large cities, especially in Europe, have specialty shops for S&M items. Leather shops often are willing to fabricate sex items for S&M people.

6. I wish to imply with this scenario that sociological interpretations of social behavior that are based solely on empirical observation may be inadequate. Rather, interpretation, if that is our goal, requires extensive consideration of meanings.

7. Perhaps the most useful methodology for understanding the nature of our existence is the analysis of personal experiences as they occur in given situations. For a discussion of this, see Douglas and Johnson (1977).

8. For a discussion on the redefinition and management of pain, as well as an understanding of the importance of the experiences of the researcher as data, see Kotarba (1977).

9. This theme is reflected in the analysis of the four volumes of *Leather Bondage Techniques,* a series of magazines that mix erotica with serious information. No author is given.

10. The norm of limits is considered shortly.

11. It is more difficult to study S&M among heterosexuals because they remain hidden. As a result of the lack of social organization, norms have not emerged as readily. One important work on heterosexual S&M is Greene and Greene (1974).

12. I do not wish to imply that the mannerisms of the leathermen are more masculine than that of other gay men; only their appearance.

13. This tendency has been noted by Townsend (1977) and is reflected in the analysis of *Drummer* and *Package,* nonpornographic periodicals for leathermen. Further, most of the erotic literature is intentionally written to titillate slave fantasies. Leathermen themselves agree that participants prefer the passive role by approximately 3 to 1.

REFERENCES

Ellis, Havelock 1966, *Psychology of Sex.* second edition. New York: Harcourt Brace Jovanovich.

Douglas, Jack D., and John M. Johnson 1977, *Existential Sociology,* New York: Cambridge University Press.

Fischer, Hal 1977, *Gay Semiotics,* San Francisco: NFS Press.

Greene, Gerald, and Caroline Greene 1974, *S-M: The Last Taboo.* New York: Grove Press.

Kando, Thomas M. 1978, *Sexual Behavior and Family Life in Transition.* New York: Elsevier.

Kotarba, Joseph A. 1977, "The Chronic Pain Experience," pp. 257–72 in Jack D. Douglas and John M. Johnson (Eds.), *Existential Sociology.* New York: Cambridge University Press.

Laner, Mary L., and Kamel, G. W. Levi 1977, "Media Mating I: Newspaper 'Personals' Ads of Homosexual Men." *Journal of Homosexuality* 3:2 (Winter).

Mass, Lawrence 1979, "Coming to Grips with Sado-Masochism." *The Advocate.* (April 5): 18–22.

McCary, James L. 1973, *Human Sexuality,* second edition. New York: D. Van Nostrand.

Townsend, Larry 1977, *The Leatherman's Handbook.* San Francisco: Le Salon.

Whitman, Frederick L. 1977, "Childhood Indicators of Male Homosexuality." *Archives of Sexual Behavior* 6(2): 89–96.

John Alan Lee

The Social Organization of Sexual Risk

The willingness to explore alternative sexual lifestyles is related to a variety of factors, ranging from the macrostructure of society to sociopsychological conditions such as role rigidity and nonpassivity in interactions (see Whitehurst, 1975). One of the most commonly noted factors is outright distrust of anything new or different. Fear of the novel and unknown is often played upon by those who encourage conformity with established norms. Conversely, the willingness to try out an alternative lifestyle may involve something akin to a religious conversion. One must "break away from the social control bind of the previous belief system" (Varni, 1973: 169).

Ironically, those who are already involved in what, by mainstream standards, would be considered an alternative lifestyle, in turn show reluctance to further adventure. For so-called "middle America," the gay subculture is an alternative lifestyle. But to the ordinary gay male or lesbian, the gay "S&M subculture" is a world beyond—often a somewhat shadowy, threatening world. Some gay spokespeople have expressed outright antagonism to their "brothers and sisters in leather." John Rechy, for example, has called gay S&M a form of self-hatred, sexism, and sexual fascism (1977). Some lesbian leaders have pronounced flatly: "S&M is a male perversion. There are no lesbians into S&M" (*Toronto Gaydays*, August 1978).

S&M may mean either sadomasochism, or slave/master. In this paper, for reasons that will be developed shortly, S&M will be taken as slave/master.

This is a revision of an earlier article that appeared in *Alternative Lifestyles*, Vol. 2, No. 1, February, 1979, 69-100. A section on the political aspects of S&M, originally included when the essay was first published, has been deleted because the topic was addressed elsewhere in this volume. Copyright © 1979 by Human Sciences Press, New York, NY.

It denotes sexual encounters in which one partner plays the role of "master" or dominating partner, and the other the role of "slave" or submissive partner. S&M sex exists in the heterosexual world, though it has rarely been studied (see Greene, 1974; Grumley, 1977; Janus, 1977). What makes gay S&M unusual is the fairly widespread existence of an institutionalized subculture facilitating encounters between those seeking slave/master sex. The institutions include bars (often called "leather bars"), baths, and clubs.

THE RISKS OF CASUAL SEX

The gay S&M world is of particular interest to students of alternative lifestyles because it provides an interesting test case for what might be called the "Looking for Mr. Goodbar" problem. Those who seek casual sexual encounters with strangers (whether gay or nongay) put themselves at risk. The risks range from ego-bruising rejections to venereal disease to injury and even death. While not discounting the other risks, this paper is concerned with the danger of injury or death.

The message of the popular book *Looking for Mr. Goodbar* (Rossner, 1975), and the film of the same name, is that casual sex, for a woman at least, will lead to terrifying situations and eventual injury and death. It would be much safer to follow the conventional road to marriage. This is very similar to the reaction of many gay men and women when confronted with an opportunity for S&M sex: "There's no way I'm going to let someone tie me up!"

When Roy and Roy (1976: 323) make the important distinction between *recreational* and *casual* sex, they identify the latter by an absence of "any depth or structure of relationship." But equally useful would have been a distinction based on the level of risk. The Roys define recreational sex in terms of a sensitivity to the partner's personal needs in contrast to sensual contact of bodies. It follows that the pursuit of casual sex for the "mere" contact without relationship would expose one to more strangers in shorter encounters. It is through depth and structure of relationships, in sex and elsewhere, that trust is built up and risk reduced. At least so it would seem, but this paper will attempt an alternative explanation.

Recent developments in social arrangements for casual sex among heterosexuals have highlighted the problem of risk (of injury, if not death). The media are reporting a new sexual phenomenon: the heterosexual cruising baths (*Playboy,* July 1977; *Village Voice,* July 1977; *Toronto Globe and Mail,* December 31, 1977). The cruising baths have long been familiar institutions in the gay communities of North American and European cities, but places like Plato's Retreat and Night Moves are the first attempt to introduce this facility for organized casual sex to heterosexuals. Every report thus far has noted one significant difference between the social interaction in the traditional gay baths and the new heterosexual baths. There is a much higher level of anticipated physical injury in the heterosexual facilities. As participant-observer Jay Scott noted, "there is no etiquette of public sex yet" (*Globe and Mail,* December 31, 1977).

The possibility of an etiquette of public sex is well demonstrated by the gay baths. Interaction is typically well-mannered and gentle among hundreds of men who are strangers to each other and in pursuit of casual, often anonymous and brief sexual encounter. Incidents of disruption are rare, violence almost unknown. In their study of five gay baths, Weinberg and Williams (1975) found a pattern of "nonabrasive rituals and . . . avoidance of hurtful rejections." Feminist author Rita Mae Brown made a disguised visit to New York gay baths: "In heterosexual life the first refusal never sinks in . . . but in the gay baths 'no means no' and the rejection is delivered without insult: No thank you, I'm just resting" (Brown, 1976).

Baths are not the only "ecological areas known as pick-up places" (Davis, 1973: 17). There are risks in a cocktail lounge when it becomes a pick-up or cruising territory. Roebuck and Spray (1967) found that the intermediation of waiters and bartenders often reduced the risks involved in sexual encounters between strangers. Humphreys (1970) described the rules and roles that reduced risk in washroom sex. Troiden (1974) studied the social organization of sexual risk in a particularly instructive situation where the risk of assault was very great. His subject was the "highway rest stop" where heterosexual truckers passing through on long-distance hauls were encountered for sexual liaisons by resident homosexuals.

A Sociological Test Case

In the course of research on the "homosexual ecology" of Toronto (Lee, 1978b) the author was able to confirm the analysis of Weinberg and Williams at six gay baths, and that of Humphreys at several washrooms. However, a more interesting case of socially organized risk in casual sex emerged than any previously examined in the literature: that of the gay S&M subculture. In Toronto, this subculture is organized around several bars, baths, and clubs, mainly for men who are interested in finding short-term (and occasionally long-term) partners for the acting out of master and slave roles in sex.

In these territories men who are often complete strangers to each other (though not to the setting or some of the other men in it) meet for the first time, go home together the same night, and act out S&M "scenarios" in which one will often become the prisoner of the other. This is accomplished through a variety of means, some rather simple and others quite elaborate: rope, chain, and locks, leather belts or thongs, leather restraints, handcuffs, jail cells, dungeons, wooden stocks and racks, and thumbscrews.

This situation looks like the "Looking for Mr. Goodbar" problem taken to its extreme in risk of physical injury or worse. Yet an examination of the S&M subculture and its institutions and participants revealed a surprisingly low level of reported incidents where anyone was thoroughly frightened or physically harmed. How do the social arrangements of the gay S&M subculture limit the great potential dangers involved?

METHODOLOGY

The methods used were those of informal, unstructured interview (except in a few cases of formal interviews of leaders of an S&M club) and participant observation. The sample consists of thirty-five men ranging in age from eighteen to sixty-two. They were recruited through personal contacts and by participation in the activities of a "leather club" in which a majority of the members were involved in S&M sex. The data were collected over the three-year period, 1975–1977.

The usual interviewing technique was to encourage the respondent to "tell his own stories" with a minimum of guidance. There were certain basic questions that each respondent would answer, but these were introduced at a natural and appropriate time in a conversation. For example: "Have you ever been really scared during a scenario? Did that happen more than once? How did you handle it? Was there ever a time when you were hurt? Did you have to get treatment? How did you get started in S&M sex? Which role do you like to play most often?"

The sample is not presented as "representative" of men practicing S&M. There is no way of knowing whether this or any other sample of homosexuals, let alone those into S&M, is representative, since no means has yet been found to enumerate the homosexual population (assuming we could develop a widely-accepted definition of "homosexual").

Likewise, there is no way of knowing the total sexual experience of the respondents. Very few could recall the exact number of times they had experienced sexual intercourse, or sexual intercourse with S&M roles. Two-thirds had had sex so many times with so many partners that they had lost count of total experiences, or specifically S&M experiences. It would certainly be safe to say that those in the sample are basing their responses on several hundred S&M experiences.

As a publicly-known spokesperson for the gay liberation movement in Toronto, a participant in the territories studied over a period of ten years, and an occasional participant in the activities of the "leather clubs," the author clearly had no difficulty in obtaining access to respondents, or setting them at ease to the effect that no moral judgments would be made about anything they cared to report.

THE RISKS OF GAY MALE S&M SEX

In any given scenario most of the risks are faced by the partner taking the slave (bound or imprisoned) role. These range from being detained longer than desired, more uncomfortable positions or conditions than desired, being subjected to "discipline" more severe than desired, and to actual physical torture.

One example of physical suffering beyond that desired by the player of the slave role was an instance in which a man of thirty was bound and then entered from the rear by several friends of the partner who played, in succession, the "master" role. Although the slave agreed to be bound, there was no mention by the master of calling upon friends (not in the immediate area at the time) to participate in the scenario.

Some men reported other less frightening events: a beating that went beyond the point of pleasant endurance, bondage in a constricting or uncomfortable position until feeling was lost in the limbs, and an accident involving a piece of unsafe equipment. It is not always the slave who is frightened or harmed, nor always the master who is to blame. No one may be "to blame." In some instances, it was the master who was thoroughly alarmed. The punishment or torture (generally called "discipline") of the slave was taken farther than the slave approved of, and the slave, in each case, rebelled, managed to break free, and in uncontrolled fury turned on the master.

In all, there were eleven incidents of physical harm requiring medical treatment: seven reported by separate individuals and the remaining four by two other individuals. Nine men experiencing injury to the point of requiring medical treatment, out of thirty-five respondents, may seem a considerable proportion. The medical treatment ranged from a visit to a doctor for care of bruises to a week in the hospital for the slave who was repeatedly entered from the rear.

However, eleven incidents of physical harm clearly beyond that which the participant *wanted* to experience as part of the sex play, out of a total of several hundred sexual encounters, may not seem so fearful a ratio. Considering that some physical suffering is readily facilitated and also actively sought during an S&M scenario, and that many of the encounters are among men who are strangers to each other — and therefore not readily held to account for these actions — a rate of injury of this magnitude does not compare entirely unfavorably with that estimated among married couples, where battered wives and battered husbands may not even have the pleasure of sexual arousal as a result of their physical pains. The low rate of injuries among these thirty-five men is in accord with other evidence on S&M (Fisher, 1973; Greene, 1974; Young, 1973 and 1975; Schwuchtel, 1976; Grumley, 1977).

PROBLEMS OF SOCIAL ORGANIZATION OF S&M SEX

Social arrangements that have enabled these thirty-five men in the sample to meet hundreds of partners for scenarios in which the men played both master and slave roles (not in the same scenario usually) with a relatively low rate of harmful outcomes of risk are of more than theoretical interest. Such behavior poses some interesting sociological questions not, to the author's knowledge, discussed in the sociological literature. There are at least four specific issues:

(1) the function of protected territories in facilitating the arrangement of S&M encounters between strangers;
(2) the screening processes by which a potential partner is selected as an acceptable risk;
(3) the negotiation of the "scenario" itself, so that the risks to be taken are clarified, and agreeable limits set;
(4) control of interaction during the actual scenario (the sex act) so that the limits are not exceeded, and real "consent" is maintained and withdrawal possible at any point where one of the participants finds "the action too much to handle."

I will discuss each of these problem areas in turn by approaching the sexual interaction in gay S&M from the point of view of dramaturgical sociology of the sort advanced in the writings of Goffman (1959, 1963, 1967, 1974).

(1) The Territories Facilitating S&M Encounters

One of the first issues faced by anyone who is interested in S&M is how she/he would go about finding a willing partner. If the intended interaction were to be heterosexual, the adventurer would face considerable difficulty in many localities in locating safe, experienced partners without incurring considerable embarrassment during the search. Looking for a regular "Mr. (or Ms.) Goodbar" for casual sex can be frustrating enough in such territories as the "singles bar." Some readers would resort to the placing of coyly worded advertisements in appropriate newspapers (see Lee, 1978a).

The gay communities of most large North American cities now facilitate the first encounters of men seeking partners for S&M sex through three specialized territories: the leather bar, the leather baths, and the leather club (keep in mind that not everyone in these territories is into S&M sex). The social organization of gay bars as protected territories has already been examined, and needs little additional comment here (see Achilles, 1967; Warren,

1974; Freedman and Mayes, 1976; Lee, 1978b). One significant observation is that the leather bar is even more a defended home territory (Cavan, 1973) than the ordinary gay bar. Those who enter without the accepted dress and demeanor are likely to be made to feel unwelcome. Leather or denim clothing is the rule, and "swish" or "camp" mannerisms are taboo. Some bars formally require a "uniform" (e.g., motorcycle, cowboy, cop, or military outfit).

Contrary to frequently offered psychological accounts of the "fetishism" of the leather crowd, the use of costume has little to do with the psychological characteristics of the participants. It serves as a means of identifying the "wise" (in Goffman's sense) and structuring accessible engagements (Goffman, 1963:195). Costume signals to those present that it is acceptable behavior in a public place to proposition another person for an S&M act. A proposition for S&M sex may be rejected by the party proposed to, for various reasons (the proposer is not the right physical type, or the party proposed to is not looking for sex at that moment, or whatever) but a proposal for S&M sex *per se* will not be out of place. The "etiquette" that makes the territory an acceptable one for S&M proposals will be concretely symbolized by the costumes worn. Thus, one of the first risks of seeking S&M is minimized, compared to what one might expect in rude or even violent reaction if a stranger in a regular gay bar were approached for S&M interaction.

If the use of costume in general helps to control access to the territory, the specific components of costume go much further; they provide the basis of a vital "information game" (Goffman, 1958: 8), which protects and facilitates the interaction of partners. The time wasted in finding a suitable partner is greatly reduced, as is the probability of miscues and misunderstandings (see Henley, 1977: 82 ff. for a heterosexual comparison).

Since their description in *Time* magazine (September 8, 1975), the key and handkerchief components of S&M costume have become fairly widely known, or at least known about, both inside and outside the gay community. Briefly, a set of keys dangling from the left hip signals a preferred "master" role; the same keys on the right hip would indicate a "slave" preference. A color code for handkerchiefs in the rear hip pockets is combined with the choice of side to add more data to the information game. For instance, a black hankie stuck in the left rear pocket signals a desire to beat or whip the partner; from the right pocket it says "I'd like someone to beat me." There are several widely standardized colors.

Men in leather bars may also wear other components of costume to further define their interests. These include handcuffs dangling at the waist, a slave collar (similar to a dog collar), leather chaps, gloves, cockrings and titrings. Even short lengths of rope or chain may be worn from the waist or shoulder (as a sort of epaulette). A man "in full gear" can be quite a sight — perhaps an amusing one, but often intimidating to the uninitiated.

An intimidating look is, of course, deliberate. Very few S&M practitioners are "taken in by their own act" (Goffman, 1959: 17). Privately they are usually amused at their own appearance and will refer to their "leather drag."

The costume signals are by no means fixed, even for a single evening. A man who spots what appears to be an attractive potential partner, but notes that the partner's signaled preference is the same role as his own (e.g., both have their keys on the left) can quietly (or if it suits his information tactics, quite ostentatiously) remove his own keys and place them at the opposite hip. He has now made himself available for the complementary role in an S&M scenario, should it prove possible to negotiate one.

Much the same sort of interaction goes on in the other two specialized territories, the leather baths and the leather club. The baths have the advantage of even more protected accessibility than a bar (Weinberg and Williams, 1975). Such baths are known among the gay communities and even their names (e.g., The Barracks) indicate the expected type of sexual interaction. Such baths also offer on-site facilities (e.g., a dungeon or jail cell). Leather clubs are frequently focused on a motorcycle theme, though many members in such clubs do not own a bike (Fisher, 1973; Lee, 1978b).

(2) Screening Potential Partners

The patrons of leather bars tend to form more closely-knit networks than those of regular gay bars. Often there will be only one leather bar in the city (as is the case in Toronto). Faces become more familiar, developing a sort of localized "face block" (Suttles, 1972). There is more likely to be a pub atmosphere than a posed and distanced one of the kind familiar in many singles bars. Civil inattention (Goffman, 1963: 83) is less rigidly maintained. Indeed, the costumes *invite* self-introductions rather than formal (third party) introductions.

The screening of a potential partner is therefore left largely to the initiatives of the individual himself, but the searcher can also find out something about a stranger by making inquiries through his own network. There is likely to be someone who knows someone who knows him. Networks tend to build up along lines of preferred roles, and to carry appropriate information for possible sexual encounters. Thus a man acquires a reputation not only for being "good sex" (or not) as in a regular bar, but also for providing convincing performances (or not) in the role he advertises. "Yes, he's a great slave." Or, "Huh, he's no master. He should have his keys on the other side, where they usually are!" Or, "Watch out for him. He gets rough once he has you tied up."

A man's reputation, built up over perhaps several years of frequenting a leather bar, and filtered through a network of friends, acquaintances, and "one night stands," may grow to include not only a general estimate of his performance, but also some details of his specialties: "he's got a fabulous dungeon in his cellar"; "he likes to be hung from the ceiling." The most important information will be that relating to the man's reliability during a scenario. Does he respect the limits agreed to? That is, as master, will he go no further than promised; or as slave, will he let you go as far as he said without complaining or reneging? A slave who "won't let you do much" is not only an unattractive choice for a would-be master with an elaborate scenario in mind; he is also a bad risk. Such a slave may give off the impression of willing submission until well into the act, and then suddenly and dangerously rebel. And there are, of course, many risks with a master whose reputation is one of not respecting a slave's limits.

Most of my thirty-five respondents definitely preferred one or the other role; only three claimed to be completely flexible as to master or slave performance. However, all but two men were prepared to "switch keys on occasion" and had done so at least once for a partner they really wanted whose keys were on the same side. The two exclusively assigned respondents (both masters) believed that it was "too risky to let a slave play the master role." This belief is not widely shared, but a modified version of it is not uncommon, namely, that it is risky to let a slave change to a master role *during a scenario*. Certainly the process of screening a partner will attempt to determine how experienced the person is in the role he has indicated a desire to enact.

If the proposed partner is a familiar face in the bar, or his reputation is known, or information has been gleaned by asking an acquaintance (or occasionally, a waiter or bartender), then little further screening may be needed. A question may be in order about the costume signals, if there is any doubt. "Do your keys really mean it?" Or, "Does that blue hankie mean what I think it means?" Occasionally someone does wander into the bar with costume he has seen others wearing, and adopted himself without learning the code.

Naturally the ordinary kind of social interaction in a pick-up occurs; we are focusing here on the special problems of risk when the interaction is expected to lead to a "prisoner" situation. The proposed partner must possess the necessary qualifiers and be cleared for encounter (see Davis, 1973; Goffman, 1963). It is worth noting, however, that the S&M setting helps to reduce the need for exploratory conversation, and moves the partners more rapidly toward the "action" (Goffman, 1967: 149ff). Like Goffman's examples of the policeman's, soldier's, and actor's roles, the S&M hunter's role is a "practical gamble" (Goffman, 1967: 170ff).

One of the objects of conversation with the proposed partner will be a determination of his concern for the enjoyment of both participants in the scenario. This hardly differs from the ordinary chance encounter with casual sex in which a woman may well want to know whether the man "just wants to get his own pleasure." But, in the S&M situation, the mutual enjoyment question is more crucial, especially for the slave. He will want to assure himself that the master is not a "real sadist," but rather a person who enjoys playing the sadist role within limits that give pleasure to the slave. Moreover, a master may want some assurance that the slave is not a "real masochist." That is, the slave will not insist on, or allow himself to experience so much stress or pain that injury, which would be unacceptable to the master's conscience, will be done. We will return to this question later.

"Promises without delivery" are perhaps more difficult in the S&M screening than in a typical male-female pick-up at a bar where a man may feign affection and commitment, or a woman physical response. In the S&M situation visible cues are available about the proposed interaction from both the partner's costume and, later, on arrival at the location for the sex act. Final screening (that is, a willingness to begin the scenario) may await arrival at the location to make an assessment of the host's "equipment." Either master or slave may play host; a slave as well as a master may keep a dungeon.

If this screening process fails to produce a sexual partner, the bar patron may resort to the leather baths in those cities where they are available. The baths have some interactional advantages over typical bar-to-home encounters.

In a leather bath a patron who seeks partners either wanders the halls, past the open doors of others, or he waits in his room for other patrons to pass by (see Weinberg and Williams, 1975). Various signals and equipment in rooms indicate the desired kind of S&M interaction. For example, a man wearing a sort of leather harness sits on the pallet-bed while handcuffs rest beside him. The visitor to his room begins to speak, but the occupant gestures *silence*. He points to the floor, and if the visitor is a novice, he may even push down his shoulders so that the visitor kneels head down. "Good. You will speak only when given permission. You will always address me as 'Sir.' You will not look me in the face. Now, raise your hands." The visitor must now decide whether to participate, or exit. If he raises his hands, the handcuffs go on, the room door is closed, and the scenario begins (see Henley, 1977, concerning the relationship between eye encounters and dominance).

Screening is much more elementary in this situation than in the bar because the bath is a safer territory than a possibly isolated or imprisoning cellar. There are other patrons just outside the door, as well as an attendant at the front desk. Withdrawal from an unpleasant scenario is possible for either party at any time. Besides, there's not much scope for elaborate "discipline" in the typical four-by-seven-foot room. A leather bath is therefore a suitable place for the novice in gay S&M to begin his career. He may also have the opportunity to study other couples in performance, since some participants get further pleasure from the scenario by leaving the door open for onlookers.

The leather club (whether it has its own premises, or holds its functions in members' homes or in accommodations rented for the occasion) also provides a safe initiation into S&M. At least in Toronto it has so far been unknown for the membership of a gay leather club to "gang up" on anyone against his will. This might be a greater risk in cities with a higher general rate of violent crime and street offences.

(3) Negotiation of the Scenario

It is rare to negotiate the actual events of a proposed scenario in the bar itself and, as we have seen, the baths make such negotiations elementary. However, when a couple who began an hour before as strangers settle the question "Your place or mine?" some negotiation of the scenario is likely—en route and at the site. In such negotiations the partner taking the master role will appear to an untrained eye simply to be dictating the script for the scenario. It would not look like "negotiation" at all. Nevertheless it is, since the slave will be responding, or not, with the appropriate cues and deciding whether or not to "go through with it."

For example, in the car or bus en route to the site the master says, "When we get there, I'll go inside. You will wait ten minutes, then knock. When I open, you will pretend to have lost your way and ask for directions. I will invite you in, offer you a drink, and then, when you least expect it, overpower you. I will tie you up, and accuse you of really being a spy. I will torture you until you confess." Depending on how well the slave knows the master, questions may be asked about the form of torture, the equipment to be used, and so forth.

This is an example of a fairly elaborate "script." Scenarios range all the way from "grand performances," lasting perhaps hours to quite elementary interactions. Thus, negotiations may involve nothing more than a simple exchange at the bar, "Do you want to go home with me?" "Ok." "You mean 'Yes sir' don't you?" "Yes sir " "Good. Let's leave now." "Yes, sir." A player eager for the slave role may even address a stranger at the bar with "Sir" from the moment of introduction.

"Scripts" in S&M scenarios fulfill somewhat the same control functions as "ground rules" in other alternative sexual lifestyles. In both cases they may be explicit or implicit (see Neubeck, 1969, and Libby, 1973: 136). Ground rules in an open marriage may limit the risk of emotional damage from jealousy and possessiveness, or even the risk of breaking up. In S&M, the "script" is almost never written, and often more implicit than explicit, depending on its complexity. It is important to note that the "master" and "slave" designations may take many forms. They may become cowboy and rustler, sheriff and outlaw, cop and crook, householder and burglar, Arab sheik and lost traveler, Roman patrician and slave boy, military police and serviceman on AWOL, inquisitor and heretic. Different scripts may call for different equipment.

Establishment and any necessary explication of the script provide an opportunity for each partner to assess the risks involved. Many players will already have "performed" some of the scripts in fantasy and/or masturbation. They will know, for example, that being tied up for an hour in a certain position is extremely uncomfortable, and more than they could bear. An indication that the partner is unaware of, or indifferent to this fact could be a warning to demur, submissively suggest an alteration in the script, or possibly withdraw from the interaction.

Either partner may suggest a signal word to be used during the scenario to indicate that the slave's limits have been reached. However, my respondents generally agreed that among experienced players such signals are rarely necessary. "A good master will know my limit has been reached without my having to spoil the act by saying so." "I know how to beat the slave so that he begs for more, even when he is pleading to be let go."

It must be kept in mind that the S&M scenario is a performance, set in a "theatrical frame" (Goffman, 1974: 124ff.). A plea to "Stop beating me" may well mean "I love it. Keep going." It "breaks frame" for either partner to have to step out of the performance role: "Am I hitting you too hard? Do you really want me to stop?" If there is a risk of the play "getting out of hand" then either partner may "rekey" the performance (Goffman, 1974: 359ff.). The master may switch from beating to the use of tit clamps until he is clearly convinced that the slave was not "really being hurt," and then resume beating. The slave may play down his protests against the beating because it is not hard enough, then "protest" more when the pain reaches the desired intensity.

Before the scenario is actually begun it will be necessary for each partner to assure himself that the other understands this process of "theatricality" and even "fabrication" in S&M sex. This will hardly be done by an intellectual or sociological analysis. Rather, it will be done by simple cues. For example, a slave who needs to be repeatedly reminded to say "Sir," or a master who overlooks omission of "Sir" after demanding it of the slave is certainly indicating that he does not understand how to put on a performance.

The successful and enjoyable fabrication of a scenario requires something of the finesse of a diplomat or an actor. The novice may begin by reading novels or serious studies in S&M (see Fisher, 1973). He may practice simple scenarios alone, for example by tying himself up while masturbating. In some cities he may view S&M pornographic movies. When he begins to seek partners, he will most often present himself in the slave role.

Gay S&M folklore holds that "a good top man (master) begins as a good bottom man (slave)." All but three of the thirty-five respondents began by a sort of apprenticeship to an experienced master. The other three were "shown the ropes" by an experienced slave. It may be possible for two novices to start out together, but this is apparently uncommon. Initiation as a slave is probably more common because it is the master who must "do things" once the slave is bound. The fact that the anticipatory socialization of masturbation fantasies would also be more convenient if the solitary player is playing slave (it would be difficult to tie himself up, then play master), may also help to steer most novices first to the slave role. In time, a proportion of the slaves learn the master's performance and find it more to their liking. However, as noted earlier, they may still revert, from time to time, with a suitable partner, to the slave role.

(4) Controlling Risk and Maintaining Consent in the Scenario

Not every slave-master scenario involves bondage or imprisonment. For example, a script may call on the slave to play the role of butler or houseboy and serve his "lord" dinner. In such instances the voluntary withdrawal of the slave from the scenario is always possible. All but five of my respondents reported that such scenarios were seldom or never performed. The preference was for situations in which the slave (whatever the scripted role) was limited in his freedom of action, either by walls or bars, or by some form of bondage. The bondage might still permit withdrawal. For example, one respondent enjoyed going to the leather baths with his partner, who he led about on a dog chain and collar. The partner obviously enjoyed this "humiliation," but could have withdrawn at any time.

The scenarios relating to our problem are those in which the slave may have entered bondage or imprisonment quite willingly, but then discovered that the "discipline" was more than he could bear. Obviously the eleven cases of sexual interaction where medical treatment was necessary fell into this category, but they were not the only ones. Every respondent, including even the two who played only master roles, reported at least one situation where voluntary withdrawal was delayed for at least a few minutes. In the two "master-only" cases the slave had gotten "out of hand" and the master wanted to end the scenario but the slave refused.

The respondents could not accurately recollect all the instances in which the action continued beyond the point of voluntary participation, but they numbered more than a hundred. In the great majority the delay before withdrawal (or at least down-keying) went only "a minute or two" too far. A master may have struck "a few blows beyond the limit." There was no strong objection to most of these incidents. Indeed, both respondents who preferred the master role and those preferring the slave role suggested that it "added realism" for a master to go just a little beyond the slave's limits. A slight amount of real fear helps to structure a convincing fabrication in S&M just as, in the theatre, a moment's anxiety that something "staged" is *really happening* can greatly enhance the entertainment (see Goffman, 1974).

Risk of really frightening denial of voluntary withdrawal during the scenario is likely to increase both with the complexity of scenarios and the containment possibilities of the equipment and the site. A location isolated from any appeal for help by distance or soundproof walls, locked chains and a gag, or a hood or blindfold are all likely to cause the slave greater anxiety. A scenario involving complicated equipment from which extrication may prove lengthy and difficult should "something go wrong" may also cause concern. Some practitioners have an astonishing variety of "abusive furniture" which they have constructed or purchased through mail-order companies. For example, there are revolving racks, hoisting harnesses, and several designs of stocks, and there are collapsible "jail cells" that will fit into an apartment closet when not in use.

A wise practitioner about to become the willing victim of such scenarios and equipment will certainly inspect such devices to assure the improbability of collapse or failure leading to permanent injury. He will also be sure that the "master" is not under the excessive influence of any drug. But a wise master will do the same, for he faces risks too. A permanent injury to a slave could lead to lawsuits, criminal charges for involuntary detention, the possible loss of his job, or at the very least, embarrassing publicity. However, while such precautions are sensible and desirable, they do not really account for the fact that, in the great majority of instances, among my respondents, the scenario was recollected as enjoyable throughout, with no point at which withdrawal was desired, or if desired, denied. How are we to account for this?

First, there are general restraints on excesses, both in the socialization of the practitioners—against violent injury to anyone except in extreme self-defense—and in the fear of consequences after the scenario is over, should either party wish to "get revenge" on the other. But, at a deeper level it became apparent that very few, if any, were "true sadists" or "true masochists" in a psychological sense. This finding agrees with that of others (Delora and Warren, 1977; Schwuchtel, 1976; Young, 1973 and 1975).

True sadism would involve the desire to hurt and punish the partner without regard for the partner's pleasure. True masochism would involve the desire to be hurt, without regard for the master's conscience or enjoyment. In the gay S&M subculture, it appears that most masters are "sexual sadists," not true sadists. They enjoy inflicting pain in a manner and to an extent that visibly arouses the slave. "Perversity . . . is where the means become the ends in themselves; where one loses sight of the fact that the goal is mutual pleasure" (Schwuchtel, 1976). When respondents reported experiences of real fright or injury, they often referred to the partner as a "real sadist." It was quite clear from the terminology used that a man setting out to play the slave role does not look for a "real sadist."

Even these observations—which are essentially social-psychological—do not provide an adequate sociological account. By using dramaturgical sociology, we may delve deeper. An S&M scenario is a special kind of "team" performance (Goffman, 1959: 77ff). The players frequently change, but the "routine" often remains the same. Instead of each player relying on the "tact" of the other (Goffman, 1959: 13ff) as a "protective practice," he must rely on the framing of the situation. This is so because, unlike the case in many team performances, the players are strangers to each other, or at least only recently acquainted; they cannot count on each other's cooperation to stage a single routine. When the partners become a "couple," regularly involved with each other in S&M, and even living together, the problem of risk obviously declines. None of the thirty-five respondents restricted himself exclusively to S&M scenarios with his "lover," though some of them did live with a lover.

The framing on which the fortunate practitioner of S&M relies for a mutually pleasurable scenario is that of theatricality. Except in the relatively rare incidents of real fright or injury, it is clear that both players conducted their performance of a sexual script as if they were in a private play. Each partner served as an audience to the other, and in the process, *contained* the other (Goffman, 1974: 135).

The great risk of S&M sex is not an encounter with a "real sadist" so much as a scenario with a psychologically normal person who, in the social situation of an S&M scenario, "gets carried away." Role engulfment increases the risk, and as Goffman has so often emphasized, role distance is the most common precaution. The safe partners are therefore those not taken in by their own act, even in a bar. As Goffman first illustrated with the joking surgeon, humor is a great role-distancer. Master and slave must be able to laugh at themselves.

Ironically, laughter often threatens to "spoil the performance" between partners comfortable with each other in an S&M scenario. The master shouts a firm command, and has to suppress a giggle at his own act. The slave pleads for mercy, desperately trying not to snicker. The presence of the potential for laughter just below the surface is a reassurance to each player that role engulfment is not threatening to break down the vital limits that make the S&M only play, only theatre.

Conclusions

The notion of sex as "play" (Foote, 1954) or as "recreation" (Roy and Roy, 1976) is not really as new as some suggest. The Roys calls it "a very recent addition to the ways in which sexual expression may be viewed" (p. 323). A reading of Ovid's *Art and Techniques of Love* (1968), first published in Rome in the year 1 A.D., or even of de Sade's *Bedroom Philosophers* (1965) will remind us that, at least among the patricians and aristocracy, sex has long been recreational as well as procreational. However, there are certainly more people who accept the value of sex as recreation today *among heterosexuals*. It would be difficult to demonstrate that argument among homosexuals, for whom sex has never had a procreational function. Gay male sex has long been playful sex (probably one of the reasons for the intense disapproval of it by those who valued only procreational sex) so it is not surprising to find a greater evidence of S&M sex among contemporary homosexuals than among heterosexuals. S&M sex is the epitome of recreational sex.

Romantic love, and thus relationship sex (Roy and Roy, 1976: 322) is largely out of place in a dungeon. The sexual theatre practiced by the respondents was not meant to be "taken seriously." The partner who is too much in love with his slave may make a poor master. He will find it difficult to fabricate, and realistically dramatize, dominance and discipline. A slave who is too much in love with his master may lose the capacity for role distance during discipline, and rebel and attack the master for "not loving me the way I love you."

There was no evidence among the respondents to support Stoller's contention (1975) that S&M sex is "the erotic form of hatred." There was no ground for concluding that those who play the master role hate their slaves, nor that the slaves hate themselves. The respondents who prefer the slave role are not taken in by their own act, and can joke about it readily. It may be that such role distance is easier for homosexuals in our society, since many must play at being something they are not (i.e., pass as heterosexuals) during much of their daily lives (see Freedman, 1971). The respondents' attitudes do not support John Rechy's argument (1977) that both gay masters and slaves hate themselves, and are merely acting out their rage against heterosexual oppression and their own need to "pass." Rechy goes so far as to claim "There is no S (sadist) in these gay relationships . . . the whimpering masochists and the tough posturing sadists are in reality all masochists groveling in self-hatred" (1977: 262).

Yet even Rechy agrees that "much S&M is strictly play-acting" and no one gets hurt (1977: 254). Kantrowitz (1976), another gay author critical of S&M sex, makes the same admission. These authors are critical of the ideological implications of S&M for the gay liberation movement. They see S&M as a bad kind of game to want to play, but they agree with pro-S&M writers (Fisher, 1973; Young, 1975; Schwuchtel, 1976) that it is a game, and that few players get badly hurt.

It is the nature of S&M as play, game, recreation, and theatre that undoubtedly accounts for the control of the great potential risks involved. Thus, similar social organization of sexual risk in the case of casual sexual encounters among heterosexuals—for example, at a singles bar—might have to await the more widespread acceptance of the value of sex as play among heterosexuals. As Alex Comfort has noted, the relatively recent arrival of recreational sex as a more widely accepted value among heterosexuals is closely connected to the availability and adoption of effective contraceptives (Comfort, 1976: 370).

The separation of the sex act from procreation increases the significance of "foreplay." S&M sex may be thought of as unusually extended foreplay. Acute genital stimulation leading to orgasm takes up only a small part of the total time and energy involved in an S&M scenario. A majority of the respondents mentioned at least once, in their descriptions of S&M acts in which they engage, that "S&M slows down the sex" or "takes more preparation" or "makes the fun last longer." The mere setting up of equipment and the application of bondage consumes time in which there is considerable sexual excitement and arousal, but no genital contact. The acting out of scripts of varying complexity further extends the excitement before genital stimulation and orgasm.

The "ground rules" of a scenario may be set up so as to prolong the foreplay as long as possible and, at the same time, maximize the amount of "discipline" to be given. The slave is thus pushed to the limits of his desired experience of pain and the limits of arousal just-short-of-orgasm.

For example, the scenario might be that of "stolen property." The script's bare essentials are these: the slave plays robber; he takes something belonging to the master and hides it well; the master "discovers the theft" and confronts the slave, who denies complicity; the master "tortures" the slave to make him confess and reveal the hiding place. This may sound like an unpleasant situation for the slave, except for the rules of the game. It is agreed that the slave loses the game if he reaches orgasm under torture, so part of the torture is the controlled use of genital stimulation (combined or alternated with beating or whatever). The slave also loses if he confesses as a result of pain. A clever slave can continue this game for many minutes by sending the master on wild goose chases after false confessions. During these respites the slave relaxes and is ready for more. Since it is also in the interest of the master to prolong the game and maximize his pleasure, he will collaborate with the slave by "believing" each confession and making another futile search. The sexual foreplay becomes an elaborate team performance (Goffman, 1959: 79).

In elaborate S&M scenarios, as in other highly dramaturgical social interaction rituals, the *raison d'etre* ceases to be pragmatic. "Consequentiality" shifts from "utility" to elegant performance (see Goffman, 1967: 167ff). Comparable examples would be a formal dinner or funeral, where the utilitarian purpose (eating food, burying a corpse) becomes a relatively minor consequence of the event. S&M may be seen as the formalization of recreational sex.

Highly formalized, social interaction rituals or ceremonies may bring together individuals who would otherwise be dangerous enemies, without risk of their even being rude (much less violent) with each other. S&M may bring together, under similar ceremony, men who are strangers and who play antagonistic (dominant-submissive) roles. Gay practitioners of S&M have developed an "etiquette" equivalent to that of political opponents shaking hands and eating with each other at a royal funeral or a political summit meeting. Breaches of this etiquette do occur (as reported by the respondents), but the social organization in which the events take place keeps them to a minimum.

REFERENCES

Achilles, N. (1967) "The development of the homosexual bar as an institution," in J. Gagnon and W. Simon, *Sexual Deviance.* New York: Harper and Row.

Brown, R. M. (1976) "Strangers in Paradise." *Body Politic* 23.

Cavan, S. (1973) "Interaction in home territories." *Berkeley Journal of Sociology* 4: 17–32.

Comfort, A. (1976) "Sexuality in a zero growth society," in S. Gordon and R. W. Libby (eds.) *Sexuality Today—and Tomorrow.* Belmont: Duxbury Press.,

Davis, M. (1973) *Intimate Relations.* New York: Free Press.

Delora, J. and C. Warren (1977) *Understanding Sexual Interaction.* Boston: Houghton-Mifflin.

de Sade (1965) *The Complete de Sade.* New York: Grove.

Fisher, P. (1973) *The Gay Mystique.* New York: Stein and Day.

Foote, N. (1954) "Sex as play." *Social Problems* 1: 159–163.

Freedman, M. (1971) *Homosexuality and Psychological Functioning.* Belmont: Brooks/Cole.

Freedman, M. and H. Mayes (1976) *Loving Man.* New York: Hark.

Goffman, E. (1974) *Frame Analysis.* New York: Harper and Row.

———(1967) *Interaction Ritual.* New York: Anchor.

———(1963) *Behavior in Public Places.* New York: Free Press.

———(1959) *The Presentation of Self in Everyday Life.* New York: Doubleday.

Greene, G. and C. Greene (1974) *S&M: The Last Taboo.* New York: Grove.

Grumley, M. (1977) *Hard Corps.* New York: Dutton.

Henley, N. (1977) *Body Politics.* New York: Prentice-Hall.

Humphreys, L. (1970) *Tearoom Trade.* Chicago: Aldine.

Janus, S. (1977) *Sexual Profiles of Men in Power.* New York: Warner.

Kantrowitz, A. (1976) "I think therefore I am." *Advocate,* December 15.

Lee, J. A. (1978a) "Meeting males by mail," in L. Crew (ed.) *The Gay Academic.* Palm Springs: Etc. Publishing.

———(1978b) *Getting Sex.* Toronto: General.

Libby, R. W. (1973) "Extramarital and comarital sex: a review of the literature," in R. W. Libby and R. N. Whitehurst, *Renovating Marriage.* Danville: Consensus.

Neubeck, G. (ed.) (1969) *Extramarital Relations*. Englewood Cliffs, NJ: Prentice-Hall.

Ovid (1968) *Art and Techniques of Love*.

Rechy, John (1977) *The Sexual Outlaw*. New York: Grove Press.

Roebuck, J. and L. Spray (1967) "The cocktail lounge." *American Journal of Sociology* 72: 388–395.

Rossner, J. (1975) *Looking for Mr. Goodbar*. New York: Simon & Schuster.

Roy, R. and D. Roy (1976) "The autonomy of sensuality," in S. Gordon and R. W. Libby (eds.) *Sexuality Today—and Tomorrow*. Belmont: Duxbury Press.

Schwuchtel (1976) (Zeitung der Schwulenbewegung), special issue on S&M, various authors but mostly anonymous. Heidelberg: Rosa Presse Verein, No. 4.

Stoller, R. (1975) *Perversion: The Erotic Form of Hatred*. New York: Dell.

Suttles, G. (1972) *The Social Construction of Communities*. Chicago: Univ. of Chicago Press.

Toronto Gaydays (August, 1978) (leaflet) Toronto.

Troiden, R. R. (1974) "Homosexual encounters in a highway rest stop," in E. Goode and R. R. Troiden (eds.) *Sexual Deviance and Sexual Deviants* New York: Morrow.

Varni, C. (1973) "Contexts of conversion: the case of swinging," in R. W. Libby and R. N. Whitehurst, *Renovating Marriage*. Danville: Consensus.

Warren, C. (1974) *Identity and Community in the Gay World*. New York: Wiley.

Weinberg, M. and C. Williams (1975) "Gay baths and the organization of impersonal sex." *Social Problems* 23: 124–136.

Whitehurst, R. N. (1975) "Alternative lifestyles and Canadian pluralism," in S. Parvez Wakil (ed.) *Marriage, Family and Society*. Toronto: Butterworth.

———(1973) "S and M" *Gay Sunshine* 16.

Young, I. (1975) "S and M" *Quorum*, 3, No. 3–4.

SYNTHESIS
DEVELOPING A SEXOLOGY OF SADOMASOCHISM

G. W. Levi Kamel

Toward a Sexology of Sadomasochism

The central theme of this volume is that sadomasochism is social behavior, which means that it may be most profitably examined from a variety of sociological and social-psychological perspectives. Rather than being bizarre or extraordinary behavior, whose meaning is accessible only through psychoanalytic theories, S&M is more fully understood by applying frameworks commonly used by sociologists and social psychologists to analyze a wide range of more prosaic behavior. Among the theoretical points of view utilized by our contributors are symbolic interaction theory, frame analysis, dramaturgical sociology, phenomenological sociology, and structural-functionalism.

Thinking of sadomasochistic behavior as a social phenomenon sensitizes us to several important issues. For example, we see that S&M may be examined on a number of levels, all of which have implications for one another. On the individual level, we are concerned with the development of sadomasochistic *identities*. On the level of interaction between individuals, we study the social construction of S&M *scenes*. And on a more abstract level, we consider the structural features of sadomasochism, which include the social norms and expectations, as well as the functions and broader implications of such sexual behavior. While these levels are distinguishable in theory, they are much less distinct and tightly interwoven in everyday life. If a sexology of sadomasochism is to serve as an instrument of enlightenment, it must demonstrate how these levels fit together. The essays in this book help to do this. They show, for example, how social organization, with its value and ideological structures, guides and instructs participant interaction during the performance of an S&M scenario. Social organization is itself immersed in a continual process of modification, reflecting the influences and requirements of the scene. The scene, in turn, is partly

197

shaped by the self-identities of the participants, as they help determine the course and content of interaction. Finally, the self is also emergent within the scene, as interaction between master/mistress and slave defines erotic identities.

Unlike psychoanalysts, who view sadomasochistic orientations as resulting from a fixation at some early stage of psychosexual development or as the reaction to one or more traumatic events, the focus among many of our contributors is on the development of a sadomasochistic identity as part of an interactive *career*. Becoming an S&Mer involves a socialization process through which the appropriate norms, values, and behavior are learned. It is the result of sense-making each step of the way, as my essay on becoming a sadomasochist and the autobiography of Juliette clearly show. This can also be seen in the Smith and Cox interview with Mistress Rose. Looking closely at her responses, we can actually see her identity taking shape within the interview process itself. As she accounts for her sadistic behavior, her definition of self as dominatrix is continually clarified and reinforced. This deepens her commitment to sadomasochism.

This brings us to another important issue: S&M is subcultural behavior, rather than just the expression of eccentric individual needs. We do not, of course, mean that individual needs are not important, nor do we mean that these desires originate solely within a social context. What we do wish to indicate is that these needs are defined for the individual by others in a process of interaction. Thus, one learns how to perceive certain situations as erotic and exciting, what roles are available and how they are assumed, and the ways in which S&M scenarios may be constructed and acted out. Sadomasochistic practices, then, are mediums of communication between two or more persons. This is made clear in "Diversity in Sadomasochism: Four S&M Careers," in which Weinberg and I discuss an assortment of S&M careers, explaining their development as the product of social interaction. The representative individuals involved came to sadomasochism from a number of directions, depending on their gender, sexual orientation, and individual circumstances. These individuals vary in the kinds of scenarios, costumes, fetishes, and sexual acts they prefer. Yet they all have similar problems to overcome including: finding casual partners, establishing satisfactory S&M relationships, and learning to recognize their own particular sexual needs. These cases illustrate one of the dynamic aspects of S&M: the ways in which master/mistress and slave liaisons are established, continually reaffirmed, and ultimately changed as the partners interact. It is this ongoing process of interaction that shapes the scene within a certain setting or social situation. This is especially clear in the selection by Califia in which she discusses how the energy flow from her slave is used as the critical ingredient in her expressions of dominance. The slave "leads her on," determining much of the action even as the slave feigns a submissive role. This, of course, suggests S&M's most interesting irony, the power of the masochist.

The norms and values that structure S&M interaction are not idiosyncratic; they are not created anew by each set of sadomasochistic partners. Rather, they are learned within a larger setting of S&M associations and organizations. Weinberg and Falk, for example, describe the social organization of heterosexual sadomasochism in a general way. The framework and functions that formal S&M groups provide to their members is discussed. In my own article on leathersex I examine the ways in which various norms, values, and meanings that structure the homosexual male subculture guide the interaction between sadist and masochist. This approach unveils the subculture of leathersex as a distinct world of meanings. John Alan Lee, in his study of the same group of people, furthers this analysis by showing how the social organization of gay male S&M reduces the physical and emotional risks involved in sadomasochism. He outlines four social mechanisms: protected territories, screening processes, scenario negotiations, and limits.

The norms, values, ideologies, identities, and so forth, in both the heterosexual and homosexual S&M worlds, are themselves part of the culture of the larger society. Sadomasochists, like all members of society, learn modes of interacting, rules for influencing the behavior of others, and the possible sorts of role relationships that can be acted out. As Weinberg points out in "Sadism and Masochism: Sociological Perspectives," the roles S&Mers choose—such as master or mistress/slave, nurse/patient, mother/child, teacher/pupil—all follow culturally approved patterns of dominance and submission. This point is elaborated further in "Sadomasochism and Popular Western Culture," in which Falk and Weinberg examine sadomasochistic themes in current movies, books, and music. Finally, as Vern Bullough points out in his Foreword, sadomasochism has a long history in Western society and has even been manifested in the lives of Christian ascetics of the fourth and fifth centuries. S&M is thus tied to both the individual and the dominant social arena of which he or she is a part.

But with all of this, one of the most absorbing questions about sadomasochism remains to be answered. This is the mystery that has baffled observers for centuries—the question of the origins of sadomasochism. No satisfactory theory yet exists.

Toward a Theory of Sadomasochism

In an age when scientific achievements offer us the hope that we will be able to understand ourselves and our world far better than any other period in history, the origins of sadomasochistic desires, wishes, and emotions are still virtually unknown. Psychologists, sociologists, biologists, and anthropologists often speculate on how these impulses develop, but they have little sound data to support their claims. Moreover, some of these claims are as puzzling as sadomasochism itself. This failure of theory is due in part to difficulties in obtaining the needed data to make informed statements. Research in sadomasochism is riddled with problems, as are many stigmatized, emotional, and highly subjective topics.

But what do behavioral scientists say about the origins of sadomasochism? Their theories typically locate the development of these desires in childhood. Sadomasochism is seen from the scientist's point of view as the result of an imperfect condition existing in the social environment of the child. This condition might be a "dominant mother" as Freud and others suggest. Or, it might result from sibling rivalries, overly strict fathering practices, or "recruitment" by an older admirer. More recently, child abuse and other forms of family violence have been posited as potential sources from which this sexual behavior develops.

At the other end of the spectrum, opposite that of behavioral scientific observations, are the speculations of many biologists. They often argue that sadomasochistic desires may have a genetic origin. Other biologists locate S&M feelings in the development of the central nervous system, or even earlier in life, during periods of hormonal production between conception and birth. Interesting as these ideas are, they are little more than educated guesses lacking concrete evidential support.

It does not seem likely that the experts will arrive at any type of agreement in the near future. This is partly due to their inability to explain the presence of sadomasochism among otherwise unremarkable individuals who often exist within widely different societies. It is this universality of S&M that is perhaps most interesting, because the forms it assumes, though sometimes different, have elements that are surprisingly similar. What varies most between cultures is not the specifics of sadomasochistic impulses, or even the ways of expressing them, but the degree of sophistication and social organization with which these impulses are carried out. While some societies, particularly smaller ones, integrate sadomasochistic practices into routine sexual behavior (e.g., flogging and biting among pre-industrial peoples), others produce specialized social enclaves. These are the subcultures of sadomasochism found in more complex civilizations such as ours.

Perhaps much of the scientific confusion over the etiology of sadomasochism would be eliminated if we had greater understanding and more agreement about what S&M actually is. This would help us to determine the structure and content of a theory of sadomasochism and what we want it to tell us. This is the first and probably the most difficult problem for the theorist. Yet, once these fundamental questions are addressed, we can discuss whether S&M is most appropriately handled as a set of desires, a set of behaviors, or both. We may then be able to determine if it springs from some drive for power, a wish for death, or some other vigorous emotion. Next we might ask how dominance and submission become eroticized. Finally, we need to ask whether sadomasochism can or should be eliminated, left alone, or even encouraged. These questions and many others contained in the sexology of sadomasochism are probably unanswerable at present, except at the level of philosophical speculation. Currently, there are as many answers and explanations as there are people who attempt them. Here we will speculate on one of the most common of these, the question of the relationship between sadomasochism and power.

S&M is a special kind of power relationship in which the master "dominates" the slave. But this is not to say, from the perspective of the sadomasochist, that power is unequally distributed. Very few people outside the reality of sadomasochism understand this critical point. *Against Sado-masochism: A Radical Feminist Analysis* (1982), a recent critique edited by Robin Ruth Linden, reflects how widespread this misinterpretation is in our culture. In this and other writings S&M is associated with genuine abuse and degradation, and is considered imcompatible with the values of human dignity and fair play. The power of submission, at least in Western culture, is rarely appreciated.

While it is true that S&M involves dominance and submission, it is seldom clear whether the sadist controls the slave, or the masochist controls the master. But one thing does seem clear, at least to insiders: sadomasochism involves a set of particular passions expressed when two individuals interact in a certain way. It is not a one-way dependency relationship in which the slave passively awaits the whim of the master. In fact, close observation of master-slave interaction might instruct the human community on how to control the hard dominance and political tyranny now gripping much of the world. Feminists in particular could learn much about harnessing the power of their oppressors with such observations. The most obvious lesson is that power relationships must be consensual—they must be agreed upon by all parties in order to exist. For a partner to be dominant, whether it be as a sexual master, a cultural force, or a ruthless dictator, the power must be delegated to him. Power will not long survive if it is seized against the will of those dominated.

Thus, if the sadist is, in fact, in control of the masochist, it is with the consent and cooperation of the latter. Sexual masochists are not likely to remain in their lowly position, and even revel in it, if they do not have much to say about what transpires. They will not stay in a situation that fails to meet their emotional needs: instead, they will modify it, or terminate it, as they see fit. It is this capacity that we must learn.

The man-equals-sadist, woman-equals-masochist equations are wrong. They are often "solved" by suggesting that women are by nature masochistic just as men tend toward sadism. These notions have their modern roots in Freud. Not only women, but also homosexual men were thought by Freud and his original followers to be heavily masochistic. But, as we have seen from the readings in this volume, this belief fails to explain many things. It does not account for the evidence indicating that most males involved in sadomasochism are slaves. At the same time women are rarely interested in S&M in either role, when compared to the much greater interest of men. Yet the minority of gay men and women who enjoy sadomasochism usually find both roles pleasurable at some point in their erotic lives. Thus, the idea that men are naturally sadistic while women are naturally masochistic does not withstand the weight of available evidence.

Even if these equations were correct, the individuals most shaken by their implications for social equality still do not understand sado-masochism. Sadomasochism is confused with the grosser social forms of "oppression," "aggression," and "passivity," as they are conventionally per-ceived. The sadist is envisaged as a chauvinist and the masochist as one who is unable to attain a higher social consciousness. Yet the evidence gathered in this book suggests nothing could be farther from the truth. In sadomaso-chism both parties hold power.

If it is true that the masochist controls the sadist through a willingness to submit, then it may also be that sadistic behaviors conceal this fact, thereby retaining the illusion of dominance. Thus, the sadist is able to remain master by suppressing the masochist's awareness of his or her power. Intentional or otherwise, this suppression may be the end product of sadistic practices themselves. As several of the essays indicate, the slave loses his or her self within the master, while willfully yielding to domination. In this act the sadist gains power.

This implies that dominance is constructed from submission, the former emerging from the latter. The derivative nature of dominance is a thread running throughout the essays in this collection. Of course, this is a view contrary to many of the currently accepted frameworks, including post-Freudian and feminist views, which see masochism as a product of sadistic behavior. Yet I argue here that the medium through which the master's dominance is erected is largely the will of the bottom. This suggests the possibility of manipulating unwanted dominance outside the erotic context of sadomasochism (for example, in the political arena) with some modifica-tion in the submissive behaviors that nurture it. This further implies that meeting dominance with dominance will not work. It will change nothing. The potential for passivity to alter the influence of one's master constitutes the essential power of masochism. Certainly this offers a solution to the many megaproblems plaguing the modern world, from family violence to the dangers of nuclear proliferation.

Yet viewing S&M merely as a power relationship between two partici-pants still misses one of its central characteristics. This is the ultimate unity of sadism and masochism. Rather than taking these to be polar opposites, it may be useful in future work to conceptualize these extremes as elements of the same erotic attitude. Perhaps sadism and masochism are not separate roles, but interacting elements of the *same* role. In fact, this is what Havelock Ellis suggested decades ago. This two-sides-of-the-same-coin view is frequently offered by sadomasochists themselves, particularly by those who insist that masters and slaves are ultimately equal. It is incorrect, they claim, to associate sadomasochism with sexism, oppression, chauvinism, and the like. It is even less correct to indict these people for using force, violence, or other means of abusing the human spirit.

In sum, masters and slaves are partners in the production of their own private reality: a reality that functions to satisfy desires, many of which are mystifying even to the participants. It would seem, then, that the more conventional members of society have little to fear from sadomasochism. In fact, the study of dominance and submission may give a better understanding of power and control, aggression and tyranny, and the ways in which persons and nations relate to one another during this perilous period in human history. It could teach us a great deal about ourselves.

REFERENCE

Linden, Robin Ruth, Darlene R. Pagano, Diana E. H. Russell and Susan Leigh Star (eds.), *Against Sadomasochism: A Radical Feminist Analysis,* East Palo Alto, Calif.: Frog in the Will, 1982.

Contributors

VERN L. BULLOUGH is dean of Natural and Social Sciences, State University at Buffalo. He received the Ph.D. from the University of Chicago and the R.N. and B.S.N. degrees from California State University, Long Beach. Dr. Bullough is the author of more than twenty-five books on sexuality medicine, science, and other topics. In addition, he has written hundreds of articles, chapters, pamphlets, and professional papers on a wide variety of subjects. He is presently president of the Society for the Scientific Study of Sex.

PAT CALIFIA is a sex educator and lesbian journalist. She is the author of *Sapphistry: The Book of Lesbian Sexuality* (Naiad Press) and has published extensively in the feminist and gay press.

CATHY COX has co-written, with Howard Smith, the "Scenes" column appearing in the *Village Voice*.

HAVELOCK ELLIS (1859–1939) was an English physician whose multi-volume work, *Studies in the Psychology of Sex,* revised numerous times over his lifetime, revolutionized the ways in which human sexuality was viewed. Ellis was interested in a wide range of sexuality, not merely in "criminal" or "abnormal" sex. Through the use of case histories, personal experiences, and the observations and reports of anthropologists, physicians, and others, he demonstrated that sexuality could be studied in the same way as other sorts of social behavior. He is recognized as an originator of the scientific study of sex.

GERHARD FALK is professor of sociology at the State University College at Buffalo and the author of nearly forty publications in sociology, criminology, education, and human sexuality. He received his doctorate from the State University of New York at Buffalo.

SIGMUND FREUD (1856–1939), the father of psychoanalysis, has undoubtedly had the greatest impact on our modern attitudes toward human sexuality. Although he did not write specifically about sex as did his contemporary, Havelock Ellis, nevertheless a concern with the importance of sexuality for other areas of human behavior is interwoven throughout his theories of human development.

PAUL H. GEBHARD is an anthropologist and educator who has been the executive director of the Institute for Sex Research at Indiana University since 1956. A colleague of the late Alfred Kinsey, he is the author (with Kinsey) of *Sexual Behavior in the Human Female* (1953); senior author of *Pregnancy, Birth and Abortion* (1958), *Sex Offenders* (1965) and *Kinsey Data: Marginal Tabulations* (1979).

JULIETTE is the pseudonym of a former professional dominatrix and madame who wishes to remain anonymous.

G. W. LEVI KAMEL received his Ph.D. from the University of California, San Diego. He is the author of scholarly articles on human sexuality. He has also written *Downtown Street Hustlers*.

RICHARD VON KRAFFT-EBING (1840–1902) was a German physician who trained as both a neurologist and a psychiatrist. Widely acclaimed in his day, Krafft-Ebing was the author of *Psychopathia Sexualis,* a work that focused upon deviant sexuality. Many of our modern attitudes toward criminality and sexuality may be directly traced to his writings.

JOHN ALAN LEE is associate professor of sociology at Scarborough College of the University of Toronto. He received his doctorate from the University of Sussex (England). Dr. Lee is the author of six books on love, sex, education, faith healing, and the Royal Canadian Mounted Police, as well as having written numerous articles on a wide variety of subjects. Founder of the Gay Academic Union in Toronto, Dr. Lee is one of the first professors to go public as a gay person in Canada. He is the father of two children and is active in both the ecology and peace movements.

LAWRENCE MASS, M.D., completed his specialty training in anesthesiology at Massachusetts General Hospital in association with Harvard Medical School in Boston and is currently medical director of Greenwich House West in New York City. His book reviews, interviews, and essays on medical and psychiatric aspects of human sexuality have been widely published, and he is the first physician to write regularly for the gay press. His most recent publication is "The New Narcissism and Homosexuality: The Psychiatric Connection" (*The Christopher Street Reader,* Coward-McCann, Inc., 1983).

HOWARD SMITH has written the "Scenes" column in the *Village Voice* for seventeen years. For five years, he also was responsible for the *Playboy* sex polls. Mr. Smith has made two movies. One of his films entitled *Marjoe,* a documentary about evangelist Marjoe Gortner, won an Academy Award. He is currently working on projects in a variety of media-related fields.

ANDREAS SPENGLER, M.D., has served since 1977 as scientific associate in the Division for Sex Research of the Psychiatric Clinic at Eppendorf (Abteilung fur Sexualforschung der Psychiatrischen Klinik). He is the author of *Sadomasochisten und ihre Subkulturen* (*Sadomasochists and their Subcultures*), Campus Verlag, 1979.

THOMAS S. WEINBERG is associate professor of sociology at the State University College at Buffalo. He received the Ph.D. from the University of Connecticut. Dr. Weinberg is the author of professional articles on human sexuality in various scholarly journals. His most recent publication is *Gay Men, Gay Selves: The Social Construction of Homosexual Identities* (Irvington Publishers, Inc., 1983).

Index